The
ROSES
AND THE
OASIS

MY STORY OF FIBROMYALGIA

The ROSES and the OASIS

My Story of Fibromyalgia

by

Andrew H. Knapp

Published by:
Winding Path Books
1753 E. 4th Street
Mishawaka, IN 46544

Printed by:
Patterson Printing
1550 Territorial Road
Benton Harbor, MI 49022

Cover photograph by :
Anna L. Knapp

First printing, 1999
Printed in the U.S.A.

ISBN 1-929080-01-8

Dedication:

To my wife, Linda, who stayed with me through these difficult times, I am forever thankful.

And to my children, Anna, Esther, and Caleb, who missed out on several years of life with papa when I couldn't be the fun person I usually was due to the trauma of struggling with Fibromyalgia.

And to all of you sufferers out there who don't know what to do or where to go, here is my story to help you find your way.

Special thanks:

To Dr. Dale Deardorff, MD, my family practitioner who truly cared about my well being. And to Suzen Alvord and Kevin Miller whose muscular and Trigger Point therapy brought me back from the edge of the abyss. And to Steven J. Mangine, Ph.D. for his encouragement and support and for the gift of the forward to this book. And to Darlene Radcliff, MSW, for her suggestions.

CONTENTS

Forward	
Introduction	7
The Roses and the Oasis	11
My Own Journey	19
Sciatica	27
Postal Stress	35
Pain Build up	39
Cheerleaders	45
Fibromyalgia	49
The Myotherapist	53
Crash Course	63
Clouded Future	71
No Quick Cure	77
Their Doctor	83
Anti-Depressants	87
The Cleveland Clinic	93
Massage Therapy	97
The Window in the Corridor	105
The Continuing Story	113
Relapse and Recovery	117
Epilogue	127
Appendixes:	
Bits and Pieces: 1-19	131
Stress	137
A Scenario	145
Some Biology-My theory	147
Muscle Memory	151
Chronic Fatigue	153
Fear Factor	155
Further Reading	157
Finding Therapists	159

Andrew H. Knapp - The Roses and the Oasis

Forward

If you, the reader, are walking the scorched path through fibromyalgia, then you probably have much in common with my friend, Andy Knapp. Perhaps you too are a truly gentle spirit, kindhearted to the marrow.

Perhaps you too, by lifelong habit, carry others' burdens on your back, without complaint, unaware of your own inner aching.

Perhaps you too drive yourself to please others at all costs to yourself, and dread that relentless voice inside, "not good enough...not good enough."

Perhaps you too are so accustomed to doing what is right, and beyond right, that bald injustice shocks you into silent disbelief, draws around you a stifling net of silence, steals your voice, stuffs it inside until the shrill protest cries out in the ache of your muscles...

Perhaps you have heard words like these that Andy heard:

"I don't know what's wrong with this guy... push him as hard as you can for a while."

"Fibromyalgia is a woman's problem."

"There's no such thing. It's all in your head."

"It's a cult. People who don't want to work have fibromyalgia."

These are words to poison the spirit, benumb, paralyze, befog, induce helplessness. Andy repelled this toxin, and found a strength deeper than the muscles, to move forward again, to learn about his body and build a new relationship with it, to engage sincere helpers, to find just work, work worthy of him. Most importantly, he found the courage to listen to the truth his body was speaking--a dark and hard truth--as his body recoiled from the injustice he was suffering. Andy shook off the net of silence--he found his voice again.

You can do the same.

And the truth of this can be bread for your journey, that you might not faint along the way. You can drink of the hope in the gentle and truthful words in these pages, the affirmation, the guidance, compassion, encouragement.

You are not alone, and the truth is mighty yet. Godspeed to you.

Steven J. Mangine, Ph.D.
Licensed Psychologist
Lexington, Kentucky

Introduction

The main purpose of this book is to give encouragement, hope, help, and a pattern to follow to aid you, the sufferer, in finding a way through a seemingly endless journey of chronic pain. Written in a play by play style of not only events and therapies as they took place, but also my thoughts and feelings along the way. Conditions and explanations of what happens in the muscles and cells of the body I have written according to my own understanding which came about through the many books I read while researching the causes of my physical pain. New research and therapies are continually changing the definitions of what Fibromyalgia is and what it's causes are, so already these definitions here are outdated. But the definitions are not that important. They are only for you to get below the surface of your condition to help you see it in a different light and find a way out. I have described the exercises and therapy techniques as they were applied to and on me, and also how I use them on a daily basis, to show that there are ways to overcome chronic pain. I have also described the difficulties I had in dealing with my employers, various doctors, therapists, family and friends.

After I had risen above Fibromyalgia to where I was in control of it, I began to meet people suffering with mysterious, chronic pain. A few said their doctors thought it was Fibromyalgia, the others did not know what was wrong with them, that their doctors couldn't find anything. People with chronic pain seemed to "crawl out of the woodwork", so to say, wherever I went. Every time I told someone why I do what I do, or Fibromyalgia or muscle pain was mentioned, they either had some type of chronic pain themselves or knew someone who did. I found myself counseling them on where to go, what to do, how to do it, there is hope, there is help, all is not lost, and, the future can be good. Often we shared tears together because "no one ever understood how I feel before".

The mysterious pain of Fibromyalgia often leaves sufferers in despair because of the absence of a clear diagnosis in most cases. For those of us suffering with the mysterious pain of Fibromyalgia, physical pain is not the only pain we experience. The feeling that no one understands how we feel is nearly as painful mentally as the pain is physically. There is also the pain, in the form of frustration, of not being believed. We "look" normal on the outside, but inside, below the surface in the tissues, is where it all lies. As you read through this book, there will be places where you'll say "Yes, that's how I feel", or "That's happened to me, too". If something mysterious is happening to you that seems to be evading the doctors, use this book as a guide to help you know what to do and save yourself some heart ache. All the things mentioned in this book have worked and still work for me. They will work for you, too. But since we are all unique in our individuality and in our reactions to all forms of stress, some things will work better for one person than for another. There is new research being done continually, bringing new therapies to help us overcome chronic pain. Try them, use them, never give up and you will reap the benefit. All you have to lose is the pain.

I am not a doctor, although I have educated myself through reading, research, consultation and hands on experience in working through my personal situation of Fibromyalgia Syndrome. Oftentimes, I don't know from where I know something or from what source my knowledge and understanding comes. As in any education, true learning is a blending of facts from various sources with experience from various sources which leads to understanding and an application of that which is learned.

For all of you chronic pain sufferers out there: Read, Learn, Understand, and Apply. Do something about your affliction. Don't let it dominate you. Stand up and take control of your own physical condition and situation in life. You can do it. The future can be good.

Come, we have work to do...

The Roses and the Oasis

I found myself walking along a path.

It was a heavily beaten, well trodden path.

It led through a barren, desolate land. The land appeared as though a volcanic eruption had rained down ash, covering everything in a grey dust.

There was no color, only brighter or darker greys.

There was no vegetation living anywhere in sight. Only a few dead, dry broken down trees here and there.

The sun beat down fiercely from a hazy sky.

There was no wind. No relief from the blazing sun.

There was no sound other than the scuffing and plodding of my feet on the path and the sound of my breathing...and my own heartbeat.

Dust rose in clouds from each step I took and hung in the air behind me as I walked.

I looked into the sky seeking a sign, but no bird of hope was to be seen, only the glare and heat of the blazing sun.

As I walked along the path in this desolate land, I felt deeply alone.

I couldn't remember how I had come to this path, where I had come from or where I was going.

I thought how strange it was that I saw or met no one on my lonely journey, seeing how heavily used the path was.

The dust in the air choked me at times, the grit coated my tongue.

I could not spit.

I was so thirsty. I was wracked with the pain of thirst. My body longed for relief from the heat and thirst...and loneliness.

I looked across the land seeking a break in the monotony, but nothing was there except for the grey hills and the sky...and the path.

It seemed as though I had been following this path for years. There was only a vague memory of life before the path. It seemed so long ago and far away now.

I came around a bend in the path. Suddenly, I detected a fragrance in the air.

I sniffed the air.

Yes! It's not my mental dreamings. A fragrance is in the air!

Hope welled up inside of me. I lifted my head. I quickened my pace. I followed the scent.

Then I recognized the fragrance.

It was roses! Oh, the delicious smell of roses. The path seemed to be leading toward the source of the fragrance.

I began to run. Although I don't know where the strength came from.

There were roses ahead!

There will be relief from this desolation.

I came around a bend in the path after a small rise and there, just ahead, was a great thicket of roses. I could barely believe my eyes. But there it was, covered with beautiful white rose blossoms.

I approached the thicket, breathing deeply the fragrance which was so rich and full. I stood for a long moment with my face touching the flowers, absorbing the delicious fragrance. I had forgotten how good it felt to smell sweet scents.

In my ears was the sound of hundreds of insects flying and buzzing amid the flowers. It was at that moment that I noticed the sound of water. The sound of a spring bubbling over rocks and splashing into a pool.

Water!

I had lost myself in the reverie of the roses enough to momentarily forget my thirst. I must find the water!

I began following the edge of the rose thicket looking for an opening to the water I could hear on the other side.

I was so excited! I knew I would not die of thirst now. It would only be a little while until I found the water.

I followed around the rose thicket for what seemed like hours searching for an opening to the water, but there was none to be found. I then realized that I had been following a path. It also was a heavily beaten path.   It seemed more heavily trodden than the desert path. A path which encircled the entire rose thicket.

In my search for a way in to the oasis, I had made a full circle of the rose thicket only to find myself back at the desert path where I had begun.

I thought,"There **has** to be an opening through these bushes somewhere. I must have missed it."

I followed around the thicket again searching more carefully for the opening that I knew had to be there.

But no.

After hours more of searching, there I was again, back where I had started.

Panic began to rise within me.

I tried to carefully pick my way through the branches of the thicket.

I held a branch up out of the way.

I held another back.

I stepped in.

I held back another branch, but then one swung down. The thorns gripped the flesh of my arm. I pulled back in response to the prick of the thorns causing the thorns to cut through my skin.

In a panic, I jumped back out of the branches to the path, blood running from the cuts the thorns had made.

I thought, "There must be an easier way in to the oasis."

I then got up and followed the path around the rose thicket again looking for anything that appeared to be a thin spot but there was no change, only impenetrable thorns.

After arriving back at the starting place again, I sat down.

Despair consumed me and I began to cry.

I was so close to the water and relief of the oasis. I wished I had never found the roses and the hope they had brought me. I had come so close only to die at the doorstep.

I looked up at the rose blossoms then down at the blood crusted scratches on my skin.

Something deep inside of me stirred.

I stood up and faced the thicket.

A mixture of desperation, anger and determination filled me.

I spoke out loud. "I would rather die bleeding to death while pulling myself through the thorns than to die out here doing nothing. I will die either way."

With that, I began to carefully pull back the rose branches and step into the thicket again.

I had only gone a few steps in when a branch swung out and held my flesh as before. Other branches caught me as I flinched from the sting of the thorns.

I froze, motionless, for a moment.

Thoughts raced across my mind. "Should I go back and search for another route?"

15

"NO!" I screamed. "**I have to get through!**"

I lunged forward, thorns ripping my flesh. I no longer feared the pain of the thorns. The fear of doing nothing was greater.

I pulled and tore myself through the brambles, my body filled with pain from the cuts and gashes of the thorns.

My body was covered with blood as I struggled on, pulling myself, not stopping until I was through. My thoughts were only of getting through the thorns to the oasis on the other side.

I began to notice a thinning in the branches. Light was pouring down through the leaves above me.

I broke through the last few thorn branches and fell onto soft, green, moss covered ground.

A pool of cool, clear water lay before me.

I trembled with joy and relief.

I reached out and touched the water with my hands. I could barely believe it was there. I felt numb as if in a daze. The water felt wonderfully cooling to my skin.

As I watched my hands in the water, I saw the blood and cuts and scratches fade and disappear.

They were healed!

I crawled into the water and rolled over, completely immersing myself in it's healing touch. My entire body was healed of all the cuts and pain and thirst of my struggle.

I laid back and absorbed the healing.

I thanked the water for being there, then drank of the healing waters.

I felt more refreshed than I had ever been in my entire life. My thirst was quenched. I was filled with a deep peace and contentment.

I made it through the thorns.

_____

*See page 135, #19a, for explanation of story

MY OWN JOURNEY

All of my life, I have been a fairly caring person. Always concerned about others feelings. It wasn't just their emotional well being that I was concerned about, but also the way they felt about me, personally. I can't say that I was a saint in this, just ask my sister, who was very ticklish and easily frightened, but it was very important to me as a life long attitude. I was easily intimidated and bullied by many of my classmates throughout most of my years of school, especially the middle grades. Disappointing my parents was a major fear of mine. If my parents were ashamed of my actions, I was devastated. I would do almost anything to prevent that. To be sure, they were tolerant of the many "kid" things that just happen in the life of every child growing up. Through this pattern of thought of preventing disappointment from my parents, I developed a somewhat perfectionist attitude. The

19

better and more perfectly I did things, the less disapproval I would receive from my parents as well as from my teachers and just about anyone else who happened to notice.

Delivering newspapers was my first job. I did it very well. Always making sure each customer received a paper in it's proper place and in the best possible condition was easy for me. Doing collections was also easy because it gave me the opportunity to talk with my customers and not be just the paperboy, but be a friend, too. Seeking approval and positive affirmation became a guiding force in my life.

Changing jobs from a newspaper route to a fast food restaurant when I was 16 years old was a real shock for me. The hectic pace which was required would not allow me to do things at the quality level I needed to satisfy myself and anyone else whom I thought I needed to satisfy. I could not perform the tasks assigned to me fast enough which caused me to meet with disapproval from the boss. The disapproval was more in my mind than the boss's, but I didn't learn that until I quit the job and went back to the newspaper route.

I could not tolerate disapproval from others. I took it personally. That I wasn't good enough. I never looked for a job at a fast food restaurant again. There were other jobs over the years that I could feel satisfied doing and some that I couldn't.

Being a Dental Technician was very good for me. There I could do quality work which satisfied everyone, including myself. I felt a sense of approval and accomplishment that what I was doing satisfied not just my immediate boss but also the Dentist and the person receiving the new false teeth. The only thing unsatisfactory about the job was the pay. With my marriage coming up, I found a better paying job, nearly double the amount, with good insurance benefits, too. The job was a struggle, though. More money equaled more pressure to perform and more speed at the task. I lasted nine months there.

At the next job, quality was appreciated there. I felt fairly satisfied with my work and approval level. The managers liked the way I worked, too. One day, after having worked there for nearly three years, a fellow worker asked me if I wanted to go and take the Postal Service exam with him. His father was a letter carrier and had been so for many years.

Now, I had never even thought about nor desired to work at the Post Office, but Bill twisted my arm and talked me into it. Good pay was the main drawing card, with good benefits and a real retirement program close behind. I took the test with Bill and, lo and behold, two years later, I was hired in at the U.S. Postal Service.

I was so excited! This wasn't just a job, this was a career. My starting pay was $3.00 more per hour than anything I had earned from any other job before.

I began on a Monday accompanying a man named Johnny on his route. He sorted the mail for his route while I went to an office with one of the bosses to fill out the many forms required for my employment. We had a limited amount of time for this and, since I always read everything thoroughly, the boss became impatient and began to verbally state to me what each form was, rather than have me read it myself, to save time. On the longest form, the medical history form, he read each item out loud to me and checked off "yes" or "no" on the form himself. I stopped him at the "broken bones" item to note which bones and at "back injury" when I stated seeing a doctor about back pain from my previous job. He asked, "Were you hospitalized for it?" I answered "no", to which he replied, "Then it's not a back injury." The Postal Service later used this against me saying that since I had marked "no" on the medical history form, I was hiding the fact that I had had previous problems with my back.

At my previous job, I had jammed my back when the fork lift I was driving, which was operated in the standing position, hit a hole in the floor causing a severe jolt to my body. The company sent me to the doctor where I received a prescription for an anti-inflammatory drug and I was sent back to work with nothing more than a stiff back. It was on my record, though, so I figured that I should include it on the postal form. The boss didn't agree so he checked 'no' on the form.

After completing the forms, I went back to Johnny's case. I followed him out to his route in my own vehicle so I could return to the Post Office after my training. Johnny was very friendly and courteous to me and all the people on his route. He had a walking route. I walked along with him as he delivered the mail and explained to me what he did and the best ways for me to deliver the mail, too. After walking with him and observing for two streets, or relays, I got to carry the mailbag and deliver a relay while he observed me. He gave me many pointers, one of which was, "Don't hurry even though the bosses will try to make you run if they can. It will only make it worse if you do." He chuckled as he said, "Just keep a steady, even pace and stick to it."

Sometimes when advice is being given, you don't know what to heed and what not to heed. In the following years in the Postal Service, I paid dearly for not heeding Johnny's advice to not hurry. But I couldn't help it, I had to please my employers.

The first 90 days working for the U.S. Postal Service is called the probationary period. It is used to cull out potential problem employees. I worked as hard as I could. I hurried to meet or beat the times for deliveries. I didn't want to blow my opportunity to be a permanent member of this organization.

When there was an excessive amount of mail, which seemed to be every day, the boss would give a carrier an "hours worth" of help to complete his route in regular time. A sub or part-time-flexible employee, me, was given the "hours worth" to deliver from that route, and any other routes which needed help that day, to keep the regular carrier from having to work overtime.

By the way, part-time-flexible meant 36 to 48 hours each week of helping the routes get the mail delivered on time, which also included gathering mail from the blue boxes around town to bring back for processing. These collections, as they were called, were done at high speed, running from the jeep to the box and from the box to the jeep, to finish on time, and were done seven days a week.

After less than two months of this hectic pace, I could hardly stand any more of it. After many, many times of the boss telling me I'm not going fast enough or I'm making too many mistakes, even though I always met or beat the times and worked very efficiently, I couldn't take it any more and came home after work in tears. I didn't want to continue the torture and mental abuse of working in the Postal Service. I felt as though I was working for the devil. No matter what I did, it was never enough to satisfy them. They always wanted more.

My wife, Linda, consoled me and encouraged me to stick it out. We really needed the money. Our second child was born the previous August and we were in the process of finishing a large addition to our house. I had no other choice. I **had** to keep going. I was working for my family's benefit, for my family's future, for my retirement. (Whatever that meant to me at the age of 28.)

The other workers at the Post Office assured me that after I became a regular, which meant that I had my own route to do and no one else's, things would settle into a routine and the bosses would leave me alone.

Well, I was encouraged and I persevered. I tried to adopt the attitude the other carriers had which was a "who cares" mentality. "Do your best and leave the rest." "Once you're here, forget it." I hated it. The money kept me there. I worked side by side with many people, including bosses, who were educated in other areas but worked for the U.S. Postal Service because the money was good, and all the while they wished they could have worked in the career of their

education.   I was sad for them and their inner
frustration.   I was the same as they were.   I was a
musician and an artist, studied in natural and social
sciences, a caring person forced not to care.   I cared
for the people I delivered the mail to.

The letter carriers were told at meetings
periodically, that only conversation pertaining to the
job was allowed.   I knew, as did every letter carrier in
the Postal Service, that I was the only connection to
the outside world for some people to see on a daily
basis.   I often was the listening ear for a lonely person
to share their troubles with or to be a comfort to the
bereaved or to offer counsel to the troubled marriage
or to share the joy of a new baby.   Every letter carrier
did these things and we were constantly harassed for
it.

Andrew H. Knapp - The Roses and the Oasis

Sciatica

I had been at the Post Office for more than a year and a half, when I began to develop a pain and stiffness in my lower back. I struggled with it for several weeks. I didn't file an accident report because there was no clear incident which caused it. I was looking ahead to a week of vacation when I could, hopefully, rest and stretch out the stiffness in my back. The vacation didn't help the stiffness improve at all, it only got worse and worse. I tried going back to work at the end of my vacation, even though there was strong pain in my lower back and sharp pain shooting down my left leg all the way to my foot, but I couldn't even reach my feet to put on my socks the pain was so strong. I called the Post Office and told them of my situation and that I was going to see my doctor that same day. The boss voiced his doubts seeing that I had just finished a vacation. It didn't really matter whether he believed me or not, I couldn't work in that condition.

Upon examining me, the doctor sent me to a back specialist. Without X-rays, the specialist examined me and, in a matter of minutes, told me that I had a mildly herniated disc in the Lumbar spine pinching the sciatic nerve causing pain in my leg. He prescribed muscle relaxants and pain killers and to do traction therapy at the hospital. I went to the library on the way home to get books about the spine and about pain so I would be able to understand what had

27

happened and was happening to me. I grew up in a reading household and was well read in many subjects including: biology, botany, sociology, psychology and several religions of the world, so I felt at home reading technical books and science periodicals.

I was to "hang" in traction for nine days spanning three weeks. Traction therapy consists of a harness, or what is called a "belly band", which is similar to that worn for broken ribs, being wrapped tightly around the mid-section of the body while lying on a table with an apparatus at the top with straps which connected to the belly band. After being strapped into the belly band, the table is raised to a nearly vertical position which feels as though one is literally "hanging" there. It is meant to take all the weight off of the lower vertebrae of the spine to encourage the discs to return to their original positions.

The physical therapist at the hospital taught me some exercises to do three times each day and some posture techniques. The most important one was the knee to chest abdominal exercise. I was to lie on my back with my knees bent and my feet flat on the floor and slowly lift my knees to my chest as far as possible without assistance and then complete the movement with a gentle pull from the hands. This was a combination exercise/stretch to strengthen the abdominal muscles and to stretch the lower back. The Achilles tendon stretch was the second exercise he showed me. It was the basic track runners stretch where you sit on the floor with your legs apart and reach as far as you can, without forcing, toward your feet. This was to be done only after the sciatic pain was gone. The third exercise was the bent knee side to side torso stretch to be used after the pain lessens to tolerable levels, too. The first posture technique was the pelvic tilt. This was to be used any time the body is in a vertical position. Instead of standing with an arch in the lower back, the idea is to tilt the pelvis forward to slightly straighten the spine to give more room for the discs to separate the vertebrae bones allowing the nerves freedom from impingement. The second posture technique was the bent knee stoop. This was to change the habit of bending over at the waist to pick things up off the floor and to bend the knee to save the back instead.

I was home from work on medical leave. Between doing traction therapy and therapy exercises, I read those library books. I should say devoured them. I became a regular visitor to the library. I read everything I could find which was even remotely related to back injuries. I came across one book called 'Myotherapy'. It dealt with the idea that muscles caused disc problems in our spines by pulling vertebrae out of align through inflamed muscle spasms. This rang a bell in my head. I remembered an article in a medical textbook written by an Osteopathic surgeon who brought a Chiropractor as an observer into surgery to show him how immovable the vertebrae are when held by muscles in spasm. It was very clear to me that a vertebrae could not be "popped" back into place without the untreated muscle pulling it out of place soon after. Many people had told me, over the course of my back problems, that I should see a Chiropractor for instant relief. I was seeking a sure and permanent answer to my

29

problems not a quick fix. While hanging in traction, I learned, not from the doctors or the therapists, but from what I read, that pressure was being taken off the spine to allow the disc to recede back to its proper place between the vertebrae.

After the seventh traction day with no real progress, anger began to overflow out of me. I was simply mad at my body that it was doing this to me. Before that I was filled with fear that maybe I was never going to get really better, like the stories I had heard of someone's friend or relative who had become an invalid because of back trouble. I asked the therapist if I could do some knee lift abdominal and back stretch exercises while hanging in traction. He looked incredulous and said that no one ever did that before that he knew about, but if it would make me feel better (mentally he meant), then it probably wouldn't hurt. Immediately I began doing bent knee leg lifts. I was in tears with desperation. There was no change in my condition after the session.

At home later, I convinced my wife, Linda, to try a technique for releasing muscle spasms I had read about in the 'Myotherapy' book where it stated that direct pressure applied at the most sensitive and painful spot in a muscle can and will cause the muscle to relax. I laid across the bed while she used her elbow, as the book said, to press on the muscles in my lower back, which were the most painful, according to where I directed her. The initial pain from her elbow pressure was excruciating and scary. Inflicting more pain than the pain I was already experiencing was quite fearful to us. The muscle didn't feel any better afterward either. We were afraid of actually disabling

30

me in using the pressure technique, so we stopped with that one try.

The next traction session began as usual. I was filled with despair that nothing was really working to remove the pain. I was filled with anger still, too. I began doing the bent knee leg lifts again while hanging in traction like before. Suddenly, I felt the pain in my leg lessen drastically. Tears flowed down my cheeks as I called to the therapists. They came running with worried looks on their faces which quickly turned to smiles as they heard me say that the pain was diminishing in my leg. They speculated as to what caused the change so quickly. They attributed it to doing bent knee leg lifts while hanging in traction. I then told them that I thought it was the Myotherapy technique my wife had tried on me last night. I explained to them what it was and they all shrugged their shoulders and said they never heard of it before. I realized that Myotherapy must be some sort of new controversial therapy which was not accepted by the medical community as yet. So I yielded to their authority and agreed with them that my success was the result of doing exercises while hanging in traction. I couldn't help but think deep down inside that Myotherapy had something to do with the reduction in the pain in my leg. I kept it to myself, though, and obeyed the therapists and doctors as the real authorities on medical issues.

I was getting better! I was going to be free of this pain! I was afraid to go back to work, though, for fear of it returning. But after a period of limited duty, which meant I was not to deliver the mail until the doctor said so, the pain almost totally vanished from my leg and I returned to normal letter carrier duty as a part time flexible sub. I had lost eight weeks of work due to the back injury, as it was officially called, but was compensated for it through Workman's Compensation insurance from a claim I had filed.

Every day I did therapy exercises and stretches. My confidence came back. There were many therapy habits which became permanently part of my every day life. I squatted to pick up something from the floor. I bent my knees to drink from the drinking fountain. I carried my mailbag cross-shouldered (which was against regulation) to balance my load. I began regular aerobic exercise in the form of bicycling to and from work. People thought I was crazy for adding aerobic exercise. "Don't you get enough exercise carrying the mail?" they would say.

One of the things I learned through my spinal injury research was that when exercising aerobically, the muscles along the spine actually lift the vertebrae slightly apart giving room for the discs to reinforce the natural cushioning effect which may have been lost through a sedentary lifestyle of constant pressure on the discs (cushions) of the spine. I figured I needed some activity without the constant weight of the mailbag on my spine.

For the moment, I had been given a new lease on life. I was happier than I had been for a long time. I was even happy to be back in the hectic work environment of the Post Office. It hadn't changed, I had. I saw the labor aspect as a form of physical therapy. The bosses still pushed me and it still felt like I was working for the devil, but now my perspective had changed.

Andrew H. Knapp - The Roses and the Oasis

Postal Stress

After three years of being a part-time-flexible, I got a route of my own. It did get a little better then. The bosses let me do my job to a certain extent. I was still harassed with route counts periodically, as were all the other carriers, and there was still the daily push to do a little more than the day before. It was still hectic sorting the mail as fast as possible and walking up to pace, and faster if many people were out to greet along the way. Very seldom was there a positive affirmation from the bosses.

With my own route I settled into a routine, actually becoming comfortable with my job in the U.S. Postal Service. Comfortable is not the true feeling for it, though. Tolerating the job is more like it. Beyond the constant harassment and nagging to go faster and work harder, there was something much more subtle going on that bothered me. That was the absence of trust from the management to the workers. They were always spying on you in one form or another.

There was a built-in cat walk above the workroom floor with narrow slots in it from which the bosses and/or agents would watch the activities below to prevent theft of the mail. Sometimes a supervisor would appear out of nowhere to walk along as I delivered the mail for a while, then disappear into a car and drive away after taking a few notes. This happened to every letter carrier I knew and to carriers in towns in different states whom I talked to while vacationing. Spying on employees was apparently universal in the Postal Service. It is good that the U.S. Postal Service is so strong on protecting the mail, but for me, personally, the constant surveillance and distrust hurt me deep down inside. I was proud of my trustworthiness. It was important to me that people could trust me and that I could always be trusted to keep my word to them. In essence, what was happening to me was that the Postal Service was subconsciously assaulting my self-esteem through their distrust.

Two or three times each year, one of the supervisors would do a count on your route. That means the boss sitting in a chair behind you as you sort the mail, counting how many letters you sort into your route case per minute, including magazines sorted into the flats case. This always included a critique of the way you sorted the mail, too. After that, the supervisor would walk along with you while you delivered your route. Of course, critiquing the way you delivered the mail while counting the number of steps you take per minute, the number of interruptions and the number of short cuts you miss, etc. At first, I viewed these inspections as a benefit to my performance and my own level of quality and personal satisfaction in my work, but after a few years of route inspections, it became more and more apparent that the process was intended to try to "squeeze blood out of turnips", so to say, rather than to be a positive reinforcement of good work. I know that there is pressure from above the supervisors to get more done, too. So it's not totally their fault.

The one route inspection I remember the most was when, at the end of the route, the supervisor informed me that, "tomorrow you will save five minutes on your route." I asked in a positive way how that would be accomplished. He smugly replied that "there are 34 lawns you didn't cross today...tomorrow you're going to cross them." I argued with him. I knew who did not want me crossing their lawns and that there were 596 lawns which I did cross. I wanted to respect their right to ask me to not cross their lawns, but the Postal Service didn't trust me to take my word for what those people had asked me to do for them. He wouldn't hear my arguments and tried to threaten me into conformance with disciplinary action. I wound up obtaining written complaint forms, after they asked me why I crossed their lawns again, from each of the 34 customers whose lawns I did not cross previously, to formally have permission to walk around their yards. Incidentally, my definition of who the customer was conflicted with the postmaster where I worked. The customer to him was the person who bought the stamp, not the one who received the delivery. To me they were inseparable. The one who bought the stamp and the one who received the delivery were equally valuable and both deserved the same level of respect.

These and other forms of harassment and the day in day out feeling of never satisfying the management made the job grueling for me over the years. I began living for my days off when I could be away from that oppressive, negative environment.

Pain Build Up

Fibromyalgia, which had first shown it's ugly head under the guise of a herniated disc, now began to slowly re-emerge as a result of the constant stress of the job. Having the attitude of always wanting to please my superiors from childhood on was difficult to live with while working in the Postal Service. Words of criticism from any of the bosses always cut me to the bone. Stress began to build up in my body appearing at first as a nagging shoulder/arm ache in both shoulders and arms that wouldn't go away. I tried switching the mailbag from one shoulder to the other every other day, which did seem to help a little.

At the time it was happening, I didn't recognize what it was from, but I recall that I began staying up later and later at night before going to sleep. I was tired, but I couldn't just go to sleep. I discovered that reading a road atlas in bed would help me be able to drift off to sleep instead of a book. My mind was always racing over the events of the day at work, the world news, or family happenings. I felt a feeling of comfort and safety when I was home with my family. It was a place of refuge for me. I didn't want the evening to end each day. I felt that the sooner I went to sleep the sooner I would have to get up in the morning and go to work. Deep down inside I didn't want to go to that hateful, defeatist work environment. I dreaded having to face the conflict and hassle of the boss pushing me each day, always defending myself in the face of criticism where I knew I was doing quality work up to my own high requirements, but almost never feeling that they were satisfied with me. The other workers felt the same way as I did but it seemed that I just couldn't take it any more.

In combination with the lack of complete rest, the build up of stress began to manifest itself in muscle spasms with an accompanying dull ache in my shoulders and low back/hip areas. My hands and arms felt slowly heavier, as did my legs and feet, with that deep, pervasive ache gradually growing stronger and more obvious. I began tripping on steps and falling often because of what felt like weakness or unresponsiveness in my legs. My co-workers advised me to file an accident report each time I tripped and fell, which was more often than the Postal Service tolerated. I received a warning from the boss advising me that disciplinary action would be taken against me if I did not exercise more care to avoid accidents. I was stuck between a rock and a hard place, between the union and the management.

The job itself of delivering the mail was becoming more and more difficult to perform each day due to the growing pain in my body. Fear for my physical condition began to occupy most of my thoughts. At times I would chant to myself "twelve dollars an hour" as I walked my route to help overcome and work through the pain. I offered the pain up as a sacrifice to God with a prayer to remove it, yet I also cried out to God in frustration asking, "What's going on with me?" and in anger, "What are you doing?" "Why are you allowing this to happen?"

During this time of growing pain and apprehension, I visited my family doctor to examine the cause of the heaviness in my shoulders, arms and legs. There was no sharp pain present. The pain was in the form of what I explained to the doctor as a deep, pervasive ache in the muscles. There was also an occasional sense of tingling and numbness in my hands and feet. The doctor couldn't pinpoint the problem at the time, so he ordered some blood tests looking for hidden infections and diabetes. This was the first of a gauntlet of tests I was to undergo and physicians I was referred to to determine the cause of the mysterious pain affecting my body. The specialists were looking for everything from herniated discs in the spine to joint problems and rheumatism to brain tumors and multiple sclerosis. The tests encompassed nearly every weapon modern medicine had to locate tangible evidence of disease. I received numerous X-rays and C.T. scans, a spinal tap, a myelogram and an M.R.I. over the span of two years. At first, I was hopeful that something would show up that was treatable, but when test after test turned out negative and the pain kept getting worse and spreading, fear began to grip me.

In the beginning of the testing and doctor visits, I kept working at the Post Office as usual, although it was becoming increasingly difficult to perform up to my normal pace due to the more obvious pain I was experiencing. It was harder to work through it with each passing day. Battling with the fear of the unknown and keeping a positive outlook was occupying much of my thoughts. I felt that my body was self destructing.   What was it?

41

What was wrong with me? There was nothing I could do to help myself. I **had** to keep trying every test and going to each new specialist with the hope (though remote by then) that something would be found that could be cured. I was afraid that I was becoming disabled, that I was never going to feel normal or without pain ever again. Life without pain was already a vague memory.

I found myself walking along a lonely, desolate path in a colorless desert.

While on the journey through the specialists and the testing, I was placed on light duty at work on orders from the doctor. Just like before, I was to lift nothing weighing more than ten pounds. I didn't want light duty. I only wanted to find a cure for what was causing the pain and to be normal again. I felt that light duty was protecting me from any further harm my job was causing me. I, my doctor, and many others, including family and friends, thought that carrying the mailbag had done this to me. It was beyond that, though.

The situation at the Post Office, however, was growing closer and closer toward animosity with each passing day. My employers were already frustrated with my physical complaints and numerous tripping and falling accident reports. The doctor's orders for light duty eased their usual harassments for a few weeks. My immediate supervisor respected the light duty assignment at first, but slowly began to suggest that I try heavier things to see if I would go beyond the light duty limitations. After many days of coercion of this sort, his frustration level reached a breaking point. I could see it on his face as well as in his words. He walked away in disgust one morning after confronting me about not working fast enough and not doing enough to carry my own work load. My own frustration was at the breaking point, too. I couldn't do anything without experiencing this mysterious pain wracking my body. I followed after him and called him to wait. Tears filled my eyes which I could not hold in any longer. My voice broke. I could barely speak. I apologized to him and said in a half whisper, "I'm sorry that I can't do this. I don't know what's happening to me." I couldn't speak beyond that, the words stuck in my throat. I saw a change wash over him, like a sudden realization or compassion, maybe. I don't know if he had ever seen another man cry before. Women are allowed to cry in our society but men are taught to hold it in. He nodded, but didn't say anything. Maybe he felt like crying, too.

More than a month went by where I was sort of left alone on my light duty assignment. I was inwardly frustrated at seeing no change in the pain in my body in spite of not delivering the mail. I stayed inside and sorted extra mail into other route cases all day instead of delivering my own route. I longed to feel well again.

The harassment did come back due to pressure that I personally felt from above my immediate supervisors. It came in the form of a phone call from the director of health services at the U.S. Postal Service regional headquarters. He questioned me for a while and seemed understanding of my plight. He asked me to put the Postmaster on the line, too. I put him on hold while I went to find the Postmaster to tell

43

him to pick up the line. When I went back and picked up the line to continue the questioning, I was shocked to hear the regional director saying to the Postmaster, "...I don't know what's wrong with this guy, if what he says is true or not (pause)...Push him as hard as you can for a while. I'm setting up an appointment for him with our doctor in Indianapolis..." I didn't let them know that I had heard that. I just quietly hung up the phone and went back to my route case without hearing the end of the conversation.

In looking back on it, I wish I had said something to ask why they would do something like that to anyone. At the time, I was afraid of them and the power they held over my financial well being. All I wanted was to feel well and without pain, to be able to do my work and live my life. Fortunately, I was neither homicidal nor suicidal, but I suddenly and clearly understood where the violence among postal employees comes from.

Cheerleaders

My body felt out of control. I was filled with deep, dull, aching pain from the back of my neck over my head and all the way down my back to the gluteus (buttocks) muscles. The dull ache was present in all of the larger muscles in my body. A heaviness, like lead weights, permeated my entire being. It was painfully difficult to raise my arms above my shoulders or to turn my head from side to side without stifling pain. Sometimes sharp, electrical type pain would course down my arms and legs. Feelings of hot or cold were present especially in my upper arms, thighs and calves. Tingling and numbness was present in my hands, fingers, feet and toes, beginning up as far as my wrists and calves, even including parts of the thighs. My jaw was continually aching. My teeth also ached. I found myself biting down hard to pull my teeth back into align. My knowledge of teeth and dental trades helped me to work through that type of pain. I thought I was developing TMJD (temporomandibular joint disfunction), along with everything else going wrong in my body.

I received a letter from the Postal Service notifying me of an appointment with a neurological specialist in Indianapolis. Accompanying the letter was a threat informing me that if I did not see their doctor they would take disciplinary action against me and possibly dismissal. I didn't want to lose my job, even though I thought it was responsible for my painful condition, so I went.

The visit with the "Postal Service's" doctor was typical of the visits I'd had with any other specialist. He reviewed the X-rays and letters of findings and conclusions from my family doctor and other specialists I had brought along. Then he physically examined me. He checked my range of motion, which was very limited due to the pain throughout my body. Then he checked my reflexes. I told him of the tests that were still to be performed from my doctor's plan to find the source of my pain. One of which was an M.R.I. (magnetic resonance imaging) of the brain and cervical spine. After the examination, he seemed to care about getting to the bottom of my ailment, though he didn't know what it was, and kept me on light duty status. I myself was getting more desperate with each negative test, though.

About a week later, I was informed by the Postal Service that I was to go to an Occupational Therapy unit associated with a large hospital in the area for testing. I went not knowing what to expect. Maybe they could help me get rid of this pain? To my horror, they only measured my range of motion and my strength levels, completely ignoring the pain I was experiencing. I told them that I didn't have to move to have pain, it was there all the time. They showed me what task I was to do and then coaxed me on like cheerleaders while I suffered through it. The problem with me, however, was that I was still in the mind set of pleasing everyone and, even though I was filled with pain in each of their tasks, I still had strength, through my own sheer will and determination, to complete what they asked.

Their findings were devastating to me. I was completely shocked. I felt betrayed by them. They could see the pain I was experiencing but chose to ignore it. They reported that I had good enough range of motion and strength to do the job of letter carrier with no restrictions. They sent their findings to the Postal Service and to my family doctor. My doctor was quite disturbed that they would ignore reports of pain from a non-diagnosed patient at the Occupational Therapy unit and sent a letter to the Postal Service re-stating my need for limited duty until and possibly after a clear diagnosis is found. We both wondered what the Postal Service had told them about me to influence their findings and cause them to ignore my pain reports.

Andrew H. Knapp - The Roses and the Oasis

Fibromyalgia

Once again I became a regular customer at the public library. I read everything I could find even remotely related to pain. This took a good amount of determination to do. Depression became an adversary. I was so fatigued. I fought my desire to just lay down and give up. Life was meant to be lived and I wasn't going to give up until I found the source of my present physical struggles. I reread some books I had read back in 1982. I read medical journals and textbooks. I searched through therapy books and manuals. Finally, in one of the medical journals, I found something under the caption of soft tissue disorders called 'repetitive stress syndrome'. This research was done in Australia. It got me excited. I had found a clue. The symptoms for this condition would not show up through the typical methods of testing, such as C.T. scans or X-rays, but only through objective communication from doctor to patient. I began to seek anything I could find dealing with soft tissue diseases. I remembered the book "Myotherapy" which I had found in 1982. I reread it. *I think I was smelling roses in the distance.* Somewhere in that book a familiar word came up. Fibrositis. I had seen it in an article about soft tissue diseases and ailments. It meant, simply, irritation of the fibrous tissues or muscles. That was it! I had found a name! *Yes, those are roses ahead on the path!*

I was anxious to tell my doctor about what I had found. So much so that I called his office and moved up my appointment date. I tried a few of the techniques for removing muscle pain I learned from the Myotherapy book, but the pain was too wide spread for the techniques to do any good. My fear of doing more harm also kept me from pursuing the new techniques. I needed something more. I needed someone who knew what to do about my muscle pain.

While at the library, I decided to try to find a Myotherapist, mentioned in the Myotherapy book as someone trained in finding and releasing muscle spasms through what they called Trigger Point therapy. The Chicago, IL phone book listed one. Hope welled up inside of me. I wrote down the number, but didn't call until after checking the confirmation of Fibrositis with my doctor. I only had to wait one day.

The Post Office didn't mind a short notice from me regarding doctor visits. I think they were glad when I wasn't there seeing the small amount of work I did while on light duty. I felt so worthless being unable to work at my normal capacity. It was a heavy burden to carry. Family, friends and relatives felt sorry for me but at the same time, I could feel the unspoken words from some of them which echoed the Postal Service saying "All those tests don't show anything wrong. What really is wrong with him? He doesn't look like there's anything wrong. Maybe it's all in his mind. Maybe he's trying to get a free ride." I fought within myself to keep the paranoia to a minimum.

At the doctor's office, I told him of my research in the direction of soft tissue disorders, of repetitive stress syndrome and especially of the word Fibrositis. I said, "I think Fibrositis is what I have." A light bulb turned on in his face. He jumped up saying, "I'll be back in a minute" and left the room. He returned with the latest medical journal he had received recently. Excitedly he said, "It's somewhere in here" as he fumbled through the pages. He stopped on a page, "They call it Fibromyalgia in here, but I think it's the same thing."

In that medical journal was a test for examining patients to find muscle spasm Trigger Points! Together, the doctor and I read that article. He followed the instructions and performed the test right then and there in the examination room. I tested out positive on nearly every spot where he touched me. The doctor was very relieved to have found what he believed to be a clear diagnosis of the source of my pain. I was overjoyed!

I was running down the path toward the thicket of roses.

I then told him of the Myotherapist I had discovered in Chicago and would he mind if I went to try it. He said that the tests we have done have all been negative. "No arthritis, no herniated discs, no cancer or brain tumor, no spinal fluid abnormalities, no multiple sclerosis. You're physically in good shape, you're just full of pain from the stress of your job. I'd like to prescribe a new job for you, but that's something you have to find for yourself. There are some medications I would still like to try, but go ahead and see what happens with this therapist in

51

Chicago." He then chuckled and said, "It probably can't hurt you any more than you already are."

My doctor had a wonderful sense of humor. As a grandson of an old world style doctor/dentist, I grew up knowing that doctors were humans just like the rest of us and should be treated that way. Not elevated like gods, but respected for their education. My doctor may be more relaxed with me because of this friendship type attitude.

The Myotherapist

From that day on, with a clear diagnosis, I felt a new freedom. The oppressive fear of the unknown was washed away. *I was standing in front of the thicket of roses breathing in the fragrance and absorbing the beauty of the flowers. I detected the sound of water splashing over rocks on the other side of the roses.* I called the Myotherapist and set up an appointment with her.

Since I was going to need to take more than one day for this, I scheduled the appointment for my long weekend from work. Every six weeks my rotating day off landed on Friday. Friday being the day off for the previous week and Saturday being the day off for the coming week. I could have the entire weekend to give to the visit to the therapist and the recovery. I had two weeks to wait.

My anticipation and expectations had plenty of time to grow. All I could think about was being rid of the pain. All I could talk about was hope for relief from the bondage I felt. I was imprisoned in my own body. I could understand how a physically handicapped person feels. I could feel their frustration, I could feel their hope for relief, their hope for a cure, their hope for anything that could help, their dreams of freedom. As the days ticked by, I am sure all of my family, friends and co-workers were sick of hearing about the appointment and all my hopes and dreams.

When the day finally came, I drove to Chicago for the appointment alone. My wife, Linda, usually did the driving because my head, neck, shoulders and arms hurt so much when I did. Linda's schedule with the kid's activities kept her from coming along. I used a semi-rigid neck brace to support my head, which helped immensely on the trip. We lived two hours from Chicago city limits with another hour to the Myotherapists office. I hurt all over, but my anticipation carried me through.

The Myotherapist was eager to meet me and help me. She said she could feel the pain in my voice over the phone. She asked me to tell her my story and of how wide spread the pain was in my body. I relayed the details to her and she beamed a big smile when I told her of my doctor's reaction to my diagnosing myself. She said, "Most doctors don't believe it if it doesn't show up on an X-ray, but the times are changing."

The next thing she did was to have me stand and measure my range of motion without pain, which was hard for me to do because I didn't have to move to have pain. I told her this. She said, "Then move to where it hurts to make you want to go no further." I had a very limited range of motion. I could barely turn my head beyond a 45 degree angle or lift my arms above my shoulders or bend forward to reach below my knees without pain telling me to stop. I couldn't (or wouldn't) drink from a drinking fountain without bending my knees. I could hear a deep empathy in her voice. "Look what the stress of your job has done to you."

She had me change clothes into shorts and a T-shirt. In the next room was a massage table which I laid upon, face down. She began finding Trigger Points and applying direct pressure to them to cause them to let go of their spasms. (Now they "reach the barrier" with pressure and wait for release. This is more associated with Myofascial Pain Syndrome than with Fibromyalgia, but I use the two syndromes interchangeably because I have found that most people with chronic pain have a blend of the two.)

Trigger Points, the way I understand it, are the center of each muscle spasm. Larger muscles can have many Trigger Points (TP's) within the same muscle. The TP is also the most painful spot in the spasm. When strong, direct pressure is placed on this most painful spot, it "triggers" a release of the spasm. The difficult part is the intense pain that is felt when a TP is forced to release. When a TP is pressed there will be pain radiated from that point to other seemingly unrelated parts of the body. For example, a TP in the scapula area of the upper back, when pressed, can radiate pain to the pectoral area in the chest. TP's in the neck can radiate pain down the arms, in the chest and ribs, in the shoulders and back, and over the head and jaw. The body's interconnectedness is clearly evident in this. I was amazed at how complex my body is.

The Myotherapist, Suzen, used her finger tips, her knuckles, the heel of her hands and her elbows to release TP's. She coached me to not resist the pressure on the TP's or tense up, but to concentrate on relaxing the muscle being worked. I can say that the pain was excruciating to put it plainly. There was, however, a certain sense of healing with it. A "good" pain so to say.

Suzen worked through the muscles in my neck, shoulders, upper back, lower back, hips, buttocks, thighs, calves, chest and rib cage, with a small amount in the jaw and face, using her elbows, knuckles and finger tips to apply pressure to the TP's. There was a continuous communication between us as she worked...

Suzen: "This is a strong one."

Andy: "Ooonn, yeah, nnngght...a little to the left, aaaagghhh, that's it, unnghht, puff, pant. I felt that one over the deltoids through the triceps and down to the little finger."

Suzen: "Your muscles are so tight it's hard to tell exactly where the TP's really are...is this one here?"

Andy: "Eeeyyaaagghht, eeyeah, that's one, nnnnghht...don't let go yet, uunnnggh, puff puff, okay,...whew, that was a tough one. I felt that one over the shoulder and the clavicle and into the pectorals."

I began to sense when a TP was letting go by the level of pain present and the change in intensity. There was almost a "taste" to some of the pain. Like an "electric" taste, maybe. It's difficult to describe, but it tasted therapeutic. After each section of the body was worked, Suzen would get me up to stretch those muscles. Sometimes stretching after a big TP was worked before the area was finished. The stretching felt better than any of the other stretching I had done before. It felt like it "worked" better. With the spasms released, the stretching became more effective. "The muscles won't stretch with TP's in them," Suzen reminded me. "We release the TP, the muscle can stretch." She told me how much it helped her when I could tell her which muscle the TP was in and the names of the muscles where the pain traveled (referred) when pressure was applied.

The knowledge of the names of the muscles of the body became a very valuable thing to have. I recommend for everyone struggling with Fibromyalgia, or any chronic pain condition, to learn the names of the muscles and the nerve paths. It will help your therapy immensely.

After giving my body a complete once over, Suzen stopped and said, "That's enough for now. Although we've only scratched the surface so far. You'll be stiff and sore from the toxins being released from the muscles letting go." She then went on to explain that the average American diet would leave toxins in the tissues when not flushed out by the blood due to muscle spasms restricting the flow. We discussed my diet next which was low in red meat and high in vegetables and fruits, low in salts and medium in sugars, low in caffeine, no smoking and a little wine once in a while. She marveled at my good diet. She said that I may not have the stiffness most people have, but that I should still go to the YMCA and sit in the whirlpool bath for an hour anyway.

My body was still filled with pain, but there was a greater range of motion, especially in my neck, and I felt "lighter" in my arms and legs. Suzen said I have a long road ahead of me to get rid of all the muscle pain and that I would probably always be using Trigger Point therapy for the rest of my life. I asked her if there were other therapies that would remove the pain and possibly be less directly painful to an already pain filled body. I didn't want something that kept me continually going to a doctor or therapist forever, I couldn't afford that, nor did I want to. She didn't know of anything, at the time, as effective as Myotherapy (now called Myofascial TP Therapy), but she had a friend who was using "different" types of therapies for his clients and that she would refer me to him when she leaves the country to go on sabbatical for two years.

I said, "What!? Oh no! I just find someone who knows what to do about Fibromyalgia and you leave the country. When are you leaving?"

"In two weeks," she said, "but don't be afraid. I have this therapy tool called a "Backnobber" that you can use on yourself. With practice, you can get real good at releasing TP's with it."

She got one out for me to try. It was an "S" shaped piece of 3/8" diameter by 19" across spring steel rod with a wooden ball on each end, one larger than the other. She showed me how to wrap it around myself to find a TP and push or pull or lean on the other end to apply pressure to release the spasm. She said to use the same count that she used when holding a TP, which is five seconds for hand, head, neck and facial muscles and seven seconds for larger body muscles. She also said to not hold the point too long because that can cause soreness, sort of like a bruise.

I quickly got the hang of using it. Suzen said, "Now don't overdo it. You've had enough for one day. Go to the "Y" down the street and soak for an hour. I'll see you at ten o'clock tomorrow morning."

I left Suzen's office and went to the YMCA to soak for an hour. My body felt all shook up. I was still full of pain, but it felt "different", like something was happening in my body. It was like a vibration all over me. I knew it was the sensation of the blood circulating into those muscles that had been in spasm for maybe years that brought on that "different" feeling.

The hot tub soaking at the YMCA felt good, but wasn't spectacular. I was waiting for the stiffness which Suzen warned me about, but it didn't come. I was thankful for the good diet I was accustomed to. I spent the night at a campground by the shore of lake Michigan. I had hoped for a peaceful walk along the beach, but it was dark and I was exhausted by the time I got there. I should have fallen to sleep immediately, but my emotions were running wild.

I had hope given to me that day. Hope that there was a future for me possibly without pain, without disability. Hope to be able to work and support my family. Hope that life could be good again, fun again, happy again, free again. I thought of who I would go to for Trigger Point therapy when Suzen left the country. Would her friend have a successful "different" therapy? If not, then would I be able to find another Myotherapist within driving distance? If I couldn't find another Myotherapist, would I be able to go back to work at the U.S. Postal Service? What job would I do if I couldn't? Would there be rehabilitation or compensation for me?...and on and on.   It was a fitful nights sleep bouncing between hope and despair, doubt and faith.

The birds awakened me at dawn and sleep would not return.   Even though I awoke with my usual muscle pain, I was pleased that I was not as stiff and sore as I thought I would be.   I was so accustomed to being in pain constantly that a change in the usual pattern was a welcome distraction.   The early morning walk along the beach was brisk, but also peaceful and beautiful. Some hope returned.

When I arrived at Suzen's office at ten o'clock, we talked about where my levels of pain were compared to yesterday. She was pleased that I was not as stiff and sore as she thought I would be. After assessing my range of motion again, which was slightly better than the day before, we started in on the session. She covered the same TP's as the previous session, but added a few more points in between along each muscle.

As in the first session, it was excruciating.   The pain being unbearable at times. I was getting better at communicating to Suzen the pain levels and nerve paths for her to follow as she worked the TP's, but there were only a few times I had to tell her to ease up on the pressure because it was more than I could stand without writhing away from the pain.

When the session was over, she assessed my range of motion again. I had gained noticeably in my neck and shoulders. I felt lighter and sort of warm tingly over parts of my body that hadn't felt warm for a long time. I asked her if I could schedule another session for next week since she was going to be gone soon after that. I wanted to gain as much as possible in lowering my body pain levels while she was still in the country. She scheduled me for the following Monday, which was my next day off work at the P.O., even though she wanted to leave that week open to prepare for her move. Suzen showed me some new stretching exercises to help keep the spasms from coming right back. She emphasized long, slow stretches frequently throughout the day. "Count 30 seconds on all of your stretches. Give the muscles time to loosen up and feel something new."

I left Suzen's office that day feeling better than I had felt in years. I was confident that I was going to get above this painful condition. I had found a therapy that worked in lessening the grip of pain on my body. I also had a new weapon to take with me in the Backnobber I had purchased from Suzen to help wage my battle against the Fibromyalgia in my body.

On the drive back home, I still wore the neck brace because Suzen said it could help keep the muscles relaxed while holding the steering wheel.

The turmoil inside me raged on. Since I felt better, would I be able to do my usual job at the P.O. and stay better? Would I be able to get off of light duty status? Could I begin to think that life can be normal again? For the moment, I was satisfied to just have less pain than usual.

When I arrived home, I gave my wife, Linda, a play by play account of everything Suzen had done and said about my muscle pain. We had hoped that Suzen, being a trained Myotherapist, would be a credible authority for the Workman's Compensation board to agree that my condition was directly related to my employment with the U.S. Postal Service. We were encouraged that she was so clear on the fact that the stress from my job was the main source of the Fibromyalgia in my body. There were very large medical bills from the specialists visits and the tests looming over us that we hoped would be paid for by Workman's Comp.

Linda was happy that I had gained in my range of motion and my levels of pain even though she still couldn't quite understand what was wrong with me. I had tried to tell her what it was as it was happening, but it was mysterious even to me, so how could she really understand what my body felt or how I responded to stress. I didn't really expect her to understand it all, I just needed her to be there and accept me even though I was failing in my ability to bring in income for my family.

I showed Linda the Backnobber and how it worked on the Trigger Points in the muscles. She was glad that I had it to help eliminate the TP's without visiting a therapist. I didn't have to wait for an appointment to have relief. It was strange to her that by inflicting more pain by pressing a TP it would make less pain afterward. It's a hard concept to understand. She went along with it anyway, though. She didn't have much other choice. It was working for me and that was all that mattered at the time.

Crash Course

On Monday I went to work feeling better physically but apprehensive mentally. Would they try to take me off of light duty? Should I try to myself? Deep down inside all I wanted was to just do my job without any problems or pain. I told my supervisor of the gains I had found at the Myotherapists office in Chicago. He was pleased but surprisingly apprehensive. He said, "Well, we'll see how it goes as you sort your mail this morning. I hope it works." My co-workers expressed encouragement and hope, too. They had witnessed my plight with sympathy and fear for me since I began struggling with it.

I began sorting mail. Confidently at first, then, slowly, the old deeper pain crept back into my shoulders and neck. I tried using the Backnobber, but it was like stopping a flood with only one sandbag. Within two hours, I was back to where I had been before the weekend. It felt worse. I felt worse. In tears I went to the supervisor and told him, "I'm sorry...I tried, but I can't do this anymore...I have to leave and do therapy until I beat this. I know I can do it now. The solution is there...I don't know if I'll be able to deliver the mail again, but I have to get well first." There was empathy on his face. After looking it up, my supervisor told me that I had enough sick leave accumulated to last nearly four months.

My words of confidence in the therapy masked my true thoughts of doubt. Despair filled me as I headed for home. How could I support my family if I have to do therapy for the rest of my life? The way I felt at that moment was far from confident. I was groping in the dark. Sure, there was Myotherapy, but Suzen was leaving the country for two years. I couldn't wait until she returned. I couldn't afford to follow her. Was there another Myotherapist within driving distance? *I followed around the rose thicket hoping to find another way in.*

I got home, shared the events of the morning with Linda, called Suzen and told her what happened at the P.O. and that I had about four months of sick leave to use for therapy. She said, "Come tomorrow and bring your wife, maybe she can learn the therapy techniques." Out of the darkness a light shone in. The thought that Linda could learn the Myotherapy techniques brought a new hope in the midst of despair and failure. Linda was more than willing to try.

The next day we drove to Chicago. Linda drove this time. She did most of the driving as I stated earlier. I used the Backnobber to try to work TP's and did stretches while riding along. When we arrived at Suzen's office, Suzen was happy to see that Linda was not a frail, petite person. "Not that small people couldn't do Myotherapy," she said, "but that it would be easier for me to teach someone who is about the same size and strength as myself."

I changed clothes while Suzen explained to Linda the Myotherapy techniques and what was happening in the body with TP's and referred pain. "You'll be learning by doing," she said. "Don't try to understand why it works, just do it and watch the results. Andy will help you by telling you where the pain is referring." Linda was receiving a crash course in Myotherapy. Also, a crash course in anatomy, a crash course in muscle names, a crash course in nerve paths, and a crash course in confidence.

It was amazing. I wish I could have been a spectator. Suzen began working my upper back and neck TP's with her elbow, explaining to Linda what she was doing as she went. As before, it was excruciatingly painful. I told her where the pain referred and she followed the nerve path working each TP along the way. She showed Linda how to find a TP with her finger, following my direction as to the precise location, then to place her elbow on that spot while holding the elbow in place with the finger and thumb of the other hand and applying direct pressure to the muscle spasm while monitoring the tolerable levels of pain inflicted on the patient during the seven second count. Linda began tentatively at first, then, with Suzen's coaching, she became bolder and very effective at finding and releasing TP's.

It would have been weirdly comical to anyone listening in on the session...

Suzen and Linda stood on opposite sides of the therapy table. Each was working TP's. The constant communication was like before only doubled.

Suzen: This feels like a solid TP...

Andy: Unnngghh, ooohht, yeah that's a good one, aaagghh pant pant blow, that one's traveling over the shoulder to the pectorals, over the deltoids through the triceps and down through the lower wrist to the finger tips.

Suzen: OK, before I follow down that line, I'll find a few more TP's in the scapula to loosen the muscles here first...

Suzen moved about an inch from the first point and found another TP about as sharp as the first one there. She explained to Linda that TP's will be clustered in some cases and can be found by sliding the elbow or finger as little as a half inch or less from the first.

Suzen: Here's another...keep relaxing those muscles...try not to resist...hold on...there.

Andy: (in between her words) Eeeegg, ooonnnt, pant puff, eeeyaaagghh, pant pant, wheeew, that was a tough one. Puff puff blow.

Linda: (finding a TP with her finger then switching to her elbow) Is this a TP?

Andy: Ooooh, aaag, aaagghht, too much, too much, puff, puff, blow.

Linda: (letting up on the pressure) Oh sorry, Andy. I guess I don't know my own strength.

We all laughed at that one while Suzen explained to Linda the way to apply slowly building pressure on a TP while observing the patients level of tolerance. She noted that my pain tolerance was fairly high.

Suzen: Your desperation must be raising your pain tolerance above the average person's range. Living with chronic pain does that, though. Let's go again...here's a good one.

Andy: Ooohh, aaeeyeah, that's, puff puff, a good one, nnnt...don't let go yet... unnngght, puff pant blow... wheew.

Linda: I think this is one...

Andy: Ooaaagghhnnnyeahnnnggnt, pant pant wheeww...

Linda: Sorry Andy, are you OK?

Andy: Don't worry about inflicting pain on me, it's a good therapeutic sort of pain...that one referred over the shoulder, through the trapezeus and the deltoids and down the arm....Oooggnnht, Suzen, you're on a eeyaaagghgood one, puff puff, don't let gonnnntt pant pant, OK, blow...that one went around the ribcage.

Suzen: Linda, let's work these points in the scapula area together to balance him out...

Andy: OK...ooogghhyou're both aaaggh on good ones eeeyyaaaghhh, pant pant puff OK...ooohh Suzen, you're on aaagghhanother one, puff, ooogh, ...Linda, pant puff, don't let go eeeyyet unnngght blow blow aaaagght wheeew...aaagg Suzen, you're on one nnngt phbbbpant pant blow eeeyyaaaggh, unnngght Linda, that's one nnooogghhtnnt unnnhh puff puff pant wheeew...

Suzen: OK Andy, sit up for a minute so we can stretch you.

I sat up while Suzen explained the importance of stretching after releasing TP's.

Suzen: The muscles need to be retrained now. Stretching gives the muscle a new boundary beyond where the spasm kept it before. Every day, every time you think of it, you need to stretch to retrain those muscles. All those years of constantly repeating the same movements under stress gave those muscles a memory. Your lifestyle has to habitually make a new memory for them through TP therapy and stretching. You need to become "stretch addicted".

Suzen then had me cross my arms over my chest and extend my hands outward. She took one hand while directing Linda to take the other.

Linda: Do we make a wish? (big smile)

Suzen: (laughing) Of course. ...Now we want to do a slow steady stretch of all those muscles we just loosened of TP's.

Suzen pulled one arm gently but firmly while Linda pulled the other arm in the same manner. The stretch felt deeply good with a light itchy feeling in the muscles of the scapula area (the shoulder blades). I mentioned the itchiness and Suzen explained that when the TP's are released, the renewed flow of blood into those tissues will bring an itchy sensation to the area. The "healing itch".

Suzen appreciated our free flowing humor. She said how refreshing it is compared to the usual seriousness of most people in a pain situation. She was also encouraged by it in that the gift of humor adds strength to the person struggling to overcome the pain and depression of Fibromyalgia and any chronic pain disorder.

The TP therapy session went on for the rest of the hour with Suzen and Linda working TP's throughout my body all the way to my fingers and toes, my face and scalp. Stretches were done after each area of my body was worked. At times the pain from the pressure on the TP's caused me to almost leap off the table, but overall, the session was extremely successful. Linda had learned how to perform TP therapy and felt that she could do it on her own. Suzen was confident that we could continue the therapy after she left the country.

My body felt warm and tingly all over. I felt lighter and alive. The future looked more hopeful now. I knew that I would get over this painful affliction of Fibromyalgia even though Suzen cautioned me to not get too excited and overdo it. The "cure" was a long struggle which included lifestyle and life-habit changes. I also knew that I had to find a different way to earn a living other than the U.S. Postal Service. That knowing kept a dark cloud hanging over my thoughts and hopes of the future.

Andrew H. Knapp - The Roses and the Oasis

Clouded Future

Linda and I left Suzen's office and went to a shopping mall in the area to take a walk. I felt better and, besides that, I just wanted to "go out on the town" with Linda to celebrate the beginning of the end of these traumatic times of physical troubles. As we walked and talked, I soon discovered that Linda was not feeling celebratory at all. The fear of the unknown financial future filled her. She didn't want me to leave the security of the Postal Service. There were no other comparable jobs with the security or pay scale to be had without the proper education and training. She needed stability in her life. Now, the stability of a regular income was up in the air with no place in sight for a landing. My ability to work as in the traditional working class family was seriously changing. Our ship was sinking and we seemed to have no lifeboat to escape in.

Linda's father was a mechanic. Through all of her growing up years, he went off to work day after day, year after year and earned a steady income for the family. When she married me, I took over as the steady provider in her father's place. Now, with my inability to work in a steady capacity, it was like her world was falling out from under her and she was scared.

My viewpoint was quite different. My father had been a plant systems engineer at a large

71

corporation. Seven years before I was born, he became crippled from a car accident. After more than three years of recuperation, he became a traveling salesman. I remember several times, while growing up, when my father had had a fall or been in another car accident to recuperate from with only meager savings to fall back on to support the family. To me, I was having a life experience similar to my own father's. I knew how he and my family survived, so I figured that I and my family would be able to do it, too.

Linda and I discussed this for the rest of that evening and into the night at the motel where we stayed. Fortunately, we are both strongly determined people. We cared for each other in spite of everything else. We also believed that God would guide us and care for us through all of this. We resolved to work ourselves through it no matter what. I think it was harder for Linda to go through all this turmoil with me than for me to live through it myself. I had to live with my body, it was just me. She had to be the spectator watching me struggle and then be pulled from the audience to become a participant in the show. I am very grateful that she was a willing and able participant.

The next morning we went back to Suzen's office for another session of intense TP therapy for my body to endure again. Suzen and Linda worked together again finding and releasing TP's. As before, it was extremely painful as each TP was forced to release. I asked Suzen why it wasn't less painful than when we first started, seeing that we had worked TP's and stretched muscles several times by now. She explained, "When the muscles have been in spasm for a long time, either from stress or trauma or both, the muscles develop habits or memories. Those habits are hard to change. After releasing the TP's, the muscle's habitual response is to return to the spasm which it has held for so long as a reaction to the stress it has become accustomed to. It takes many, many TP releases with stretching and lifestyle changes to replace the old muscle response habit memory with a new muscle response habit memory." She then said, "I hate to tell you this, but you have a lifetime ahead of you of working TP's and stretching and re-educating your muscles."

I understood immediately as soon as Suzen mentioned muscle memory and habitual responses. "So", I said, "you mean there's no cure for this Fibromyalgia? I've got to struggle with this forever?" Linda echoed my questions. Suzen assured us that we could and would get above it but that it would take a constant vigilance to rise above it and stay above it. It would take definite lifestyle changes, which meant many things, the biggest of which was a new way to earn a living which did not have the high stress levels like my present employer, the U.S. Postal Service.

I began to run with the idea. I mentioned that I could change some muscle habits by switching hands from right handed to left handed on things which I usually do, such as eating or brushing my teeth or drying my back with the towel over the opposite shoulder or anything that was a deep muscle habit. I had already been doing that more than a year previous by sorting the mail with the left hand rather the right and by delivering the mail with the mailbag over the opposite shoulder and placing mail into home receptacles with the left hand, too. I stated to Suzen that I noticed no real lessening of the pain levels by doing that, but that it seemed that there wouldn't be any difference from switching hands or stretching or even an elimination of stress sources without releasing the muscle spasms first. Suzen marveled at my understanding of how it all worked together. She concurred that I could stretch and stretch and do exercises after exercises and maybe improve a little but never rise above it until the muscles were cleared of spasms and TP's.

Tears filled my eyes again. I said, "Well, let's keep going then. All I want is to be free again." Suzen and Linda continued to inflict the healing pain of the TP and spasm release therapy to the muscles of my body. I endured it with the deeply satisfying knowing that eventually I would rise above it to live life without pain inhibiting my every move.

After the session was over, I asked Suzen to write a short explanation of my condition of Fibromyalgia and of my job environment which was the major cause of it for me. She said that she would be happy to do that for me but her word would not be good enough for any legal case because she was not a doctor, especially when dealing with such a large organization as the U.S. Postal Service. She was just a Myotherapist.

She did write up something and sent it with us saying, "Even if they don't consider my authority worth anything, put this in beside your doctor's affidavit. Two letters agreeing on a cause will hopefully shed some light into what really happens

74

inside the Postal Service which causes so many problems with their employees. All you can do is try." She paused and then said, "Truthfully, your case is a tough one because your job, your work, isn't the only thing that has done this to you. It's the stress of your job that has caused you to develop Fibromyalgia. It's not the just the physical work, it's the stress and how you cope or not cope with it. It's not tangible, it's on an objective level and not clearly provable. I'm sure that's what they'll aim at in their own defense. Hopefully, Workman's Comp. will pay for the tests and doctor visits. But first and most importantly, you need to concentrate on getting yourself physically better. After that you can look for another less stressful career. Look for something in music or science, things that you enjoy doing, then Fibromyalgia won't be as much of a hindrance to you...You can do it. You'll look back on this and be thankful that it gave you the opportunity to find a different career."

Linda and I were encouraged by Suzen's words. We knew we were in for a struggle in the coming years, but all we could do was to get past the troubles of the moment. The future was a topic of speculation and a source of worry which I didn't need but couldn't escape from. We left Suzen's office that day filled with a wide range of emotion ranging from exhilaration at finding a way to treat my physical pain to a heavy sort of depression from the uncertain future ahead of us.

Andrew H. Knapp - The Roses and the Oasis

No Quick Cure

The following week was a roller coaster for us to put it mildly. First, I consulted with my personal doctor and shared with him the play by play of the therapy sessions with Suzen and that Linda had learned how to administer the therapy. He beamed with delight and happiness for me that finally something was going my way. He said that he had some medications for me to try someday which he thought might be worthwhile. He wanted to give the Myotherapy a month or so to see how well it works before prescribing any of the new medications. The same week, I received a letter from the U.S. Postal Service informing me of an appointment with their doctor in Indianapolis again. I was actually rather eager to see him now that I had a clear diagnosis and an effective therapy to boot. I should have known better, though.

The appointment was set up for a month from that date. I was to bring all updated X-rays and test results along with me. Just thinking about the U.S. Postal Service caused my body to tense up. I didn't want to go back to that place. I didn't want to enter that stress filled environment again.

Every day, Linda performed Myotherapy on my body. I did stretches and used the Backnobber many times each day. I was gaining in lowering the pain levels and improving my pain free range of motion. I still had pain and stiffness, but I was seeing improvement.

After two weeks, I wondered what new ideas the other therapist in Chicago, which Suzen had suggested me to try, too, might have to add to my success. I called him and set up an appointment for the next week, four days before the Indianapolis appointment.

It was now summer break from school for the kids, so we all made the trip to Chicago together. Linda and the kids went to the Aquarium while I went to the therapist. He was a fairly friendly person, though he regarded Suzen's Myotherapy techniques as rather "barbaric". It was quite apparent that she thought more of him than he thought of her. He began by my giving him a short history of my struggle with Fibromyalgia pain and then checked my range of motion. He asked me how far I could move my head from side to side. I moved my head to one side and stopped where the pain began to intensify. I said, "Unnghh, it hurts pretty bad here, but,"...I then turned my head to nearly 90 degrees..."I can go, unnhhh, all the way to here, nnnggghht, puff whew." He looked incredulous. "Why would you go past where the pain gets bad?" He nearly shouted those words. "I've never had a patient who would move beyond where it hurts."

I thought for a moment about his question of why. I suddenly recalled my father who had been crippled from car accidents. I remembered that much of the time when he reached for something he would get part way there, groan or grimace with pain, then complete the movement to reach what he wanted to pick up. I grew up seeing that example of how to deal with pain. I shared all of this with the therapist.

The therapist exclaimed, "No wonder the Postal Service doesn't believe you! You can force yourself through pain! Your pain must have been extreme for you to even seek help at all."

My thoughts raced. It all made sense as to how Fibromyalgia would build up in my body realizing my attitude toward dealing with pain. The way I cared and empathized with other peoples needs, never wanting to cause anyone extra work or effort or worry because of me. If I stopped forcing myself through pain now, at this point, I would become an invalid. I would never get ahead of the pain levels without working through it. If my father had stopped trying when it hurt, he would have become completely helpless. He never lost his dignity through it all. I felt proud of him in a way I had not felt before. He had worked through it and so would I.

The therapist examined my spine and body alignment after my range of motion display. He noticed two vertebrae were out of align. One in the neck and one in the center of my back. He asked if I had ever had any spinal manipulation done before, which meant, had anyone popped my spine back into place as chiropractors do. I said no to which he asked would I mind if he re-aligned the two out of place vertebrae in my spine for me now. Having never had it done before, I said, "Why not? There's not much to lose, let's go for it." While he was getting me into position, I relayed to him my knowledge of the muscles of the body being able to pull vertebrae out of align and that if the muscles were in spasm, wouldn't the vertebrae be pulled back out of align soon after being popped into place? He simply said, "Hmm, I suppose it could. It may help, though. Do you still want to try it?" I said OK and he first popped my neck with a quick jerk sideways to my head. I felt a deep pop in my spine there. It gave me a sort of funny, strange, feeling in that spot for a few minutes, which actually lingered for a few hours afterward. He then popped my middle spine vertebrae back into place by having me hold one of my arms over my head and, with both of his arms around my upper body, jerked me somehow causing another heavy pop deep inside of my body. A strange sort of heaviness permeated my being from those two pops. It had a "doesn't feel right" sense deep within. The therapist had me do a few stretches and checked my range of motion again. It was basically the same as before to which he said that I should keep stretching. I didn't say it, but I knew that if I only stretched the muscles without releasing spasms, the muscles would pull the vertebrae back out of align again.

He examined my feet next. He noticed that my second toe on each foot was slightly longer than the big toe. They looked quite close to the same length to me, but yes, the second toe was longer. As he pointed this out to me he explained that people who have LST (long second toe) have a tendency to develop pain in their feet because the second toe joint has more pressure applied to it from walking, running or standing than the other smaller toes. This causes a strain on the tendons in the middle of the foot. I mentioned to him that Suzen, the Myotherapist, had noticed it and had given me some small felt inserts to place under the big toe ball to alleviate pressure on the second toe joint. She said that her therapist friend told her about it and he says that it helps many of his clients. I knew that this was her therapist friend. At this point, I began to respect his authority less and less because I could see that he was searching for any mysterious thing that could cause pain in the body and that he didn't want to continue the success I had experienced with Trigger Point therapy even though I wanted him to. He apparently didn't know how or didn't believe that it worked. I knew I was being a difficult patient, but I was no longer aimless in my search for help. I knew what was causing the pain in my muscles and had already found a therapy that brought some relief and change in my condition. I knew that the source of the pain in my feet was from further up in my body along the nerve path in muscles in my legs, buttocks and back and not in the tendons in my feet. Anatomically and biologically Trigger Point therapy made complete sense.

I questioned this tendon strain idea. He acknowledged my rational thinking and said, "Well, if the felt toe inserts bring more comfort, then it's worth a try." I went along with that then.

Next he asked about my teeth and the amount of filling material I had in them. There was plenty. Having grown up without much dental hygiene practices in the 50's and early 60's, I had large fillings in most of my teeth. He began talking about mercury poisoning, which affects the nerves of the body, from the mercury used to soften the silver for application in fillings in teeth.

My skepticism of his practices began to surface. I knew that the mercury became chemically stable after solidifying with the silver. He said that the filings from scraping the fillings to make them fit into the cavity holes may have been ingested causing a build up of toxic mercury in the tissues. Over the years and many fillings, you could develop a toxic build up bringing about a reaction in your body. We discussed this since I openly disagreed with him. I had already gone over the effects of toxic heavy metal build up in the body as well as other non metal toxins in my research to discover the source of my muscle pain afflictions. He was obviously uncomfortable with my knowledge of the causes of painful conditions in the body. I was disappointed in him. He seemed to be like many of the doctors I had visited who were looking for a quick, instant fix of my problem such as surgery or the latest pill or some spinal manipulation "pops". It was becoming more and more obvious that there was no magical cure for Fibromyalgia. There was just determination and work ahead for me.

I left the therapists office that day feeling strangely uncomfortable deep inside from the two spinal manipulations he had administered and from the feeling that I had wasted my time and money there. The feeling from the spinal manipulation did go away later that day, but there was no change like the "quick cure" it was supposed to be.

Their Doctor

My next hurdle to cross was the second visit with the specialist in Indianapolis hired by the Postal Service. Now that I had a clear diagnosis of Fibromyalgia, I was eager to see him and share with him the success in treating it with TP therapy so far. The visit was the same situation as the second therapist in Chicago. The whole family went down together. Linda drove while I wore the neck brace and did TP therapy with the Backnobber on various muscles in my body and the kids rode along enjoying the ride.

I must mention that fatigue was a major hindrance in doing the therapy on myself as well as for doing anything at all. My body was constantly fighting the pain from the Fibromyalgia and also enduring the TP therapy pain at the same time. This constant fighting of pain sapped a great deal of energy from me. My own determination to defeat Fibromyalgia was what kept me going. I continually fought my natural inclination to lay down, rest and do nothing. This inclination however, would never stop the pain-causing muscle spasms which kept me in pain even while sleeping and resting. The fear of my unknown future still added to the tendency my body had developed to tense the muscles when dealing with stress.

We arrived at the doctor's office and were cordially greeted by him. He himself offered lollipops to my three children. I then followed him back to one of the examining rooms. I handed him the packet of X-rays and test results which included the letter from Suzen, the Myotherapist. He placed them aside without even looking at them. I had removed the neck brace earlier and carried it in along with the X-rays. He seemed apprehensive about something, then he asked me to remove my shirt so he could check my range of motion. I performed the whole range of motion exam telling when the pain intensified and then began telling him of the Fibromyalgia diagnosis and the discovery of TP therapy which was giving some success in reducing some of the pain levels. He became very curt and blunt with me then. "Fibromyalgia is a woman's problem," he said. "There's no such thing. It's all in your head. There's nothing wrong with you. Go back to work." I argued with him, defending myself and the mysterious way in which this Fibromyalgia ailment had come and gotten me and how my own doctor and the Myotherapist could attest to the validity of my situation. He wouldn't listen to me. He looked me square in the eye and said rather angrily, "Some of us don't believe in this stress sort of thing. It's a cult. People who don't want to work have Fibromyalgia." He looked away and then back. "Like I just said, go back to work, there's nothing wrong with you. It's all in your head." He reached for the door, "Put your shirt back on, we're done." I followed him out of the room without my shirt pleading with him to listen to the authorities who have done the research. He simply restated himself, "Some of us just don't believe in this sort of thing. You need to go back to work."

I was completely in shock. I understood more clearly than before why there are killings and suicides among employees of the U.S. Postal Service. My non-violent nature, coupled with my compassion for him above his errant ways, kept another violent postal worker outburst from happening. I realized that this doctor was hired by the Postal Service and would diagnose with a bias toward the system and not follow the Hippocratic oath in some cases.

I pulled myself away from him and went back to the room to get my shirt and X-ray packet. It was obvious to me that his response was pre-meditated with no concern for my physical state. I don't remember ever being as angry as I was at that moment before in my life. I was angry at the gross injustice which was just handed to me. The doctor was only the puppet through which it was delivered.

My anger, shock and bewilderment kept the tears from flowing that day. I felt chewed up and spat out by the U.S.P.S. I had been used, abused and discarded. The U.S. Postal Service was completely against me, there was no compassion there. As the superiors and bosses say, "I hate to do this, but it's my job." Harass and manipulate all in the name of earning money. I felt betrayed. I naively trusted my employer to help me through my physical troubles, but no, I was a financial burden to them. I was costing them money. I was expendable.

We left the doctor's office and went to the Children's Museum where I tried to lose myself in the fun the kids were having. My body was all tensed up with muscle spasms filling my body with renewed pain. The episode with that doctor caused a major relapse of pain in muscles which had shown definite improvement before. It seemed that every time I had to communicate directly with the Postal Service I would suffer an increase in pain levels in my body from the stress of the encounter. Sort of like having to deal with a class bully every day with the fear of being beaten for no reason even if I was real nice.

Anti-Depressants

On the way home, while the kids were sleeping, Linda and I shared my despair and tried to paint a hopeful future. We decided that after I got to a level of manageable pain, I could advertise more for performances, which had the potential of a very good income, and look for a booking agent then, too. It was very clear that the Postal Service was out of the question due to the intolerable stress levels for me there. I could look into other trades in the music industry such as musical instrument repair or giving lessons. I played several instruments well. With a good clientele I could make a comfortable living. Linda could get a part time job, ideally working in the school system, where she could be home when the kids were there.

We slowly began to realize that there were other ways to make a living besides the Postal Service. The steady work and income of the Postal Service had spoiled us to the point of dependency on a certain lifestyle and economic level. We were afraid to set out in our own little boat after being used to the luxury of an ocean liner even though we were only deck hands who were not meant to enjoy the cruise. We concluded that life was becoming an adventure for us. I knew that my folks had made it, even though it was fairly meager for them. I was

87

determined to make it through this and to make it better than my parents did.

Shortly after returning from Indianapolis, I put together a mailing for my performances at schools. I sent nearly 500 brochures to area elementary schools within a 150 mile radius of home. Soon I began to receive calls for bookings. It was encouraging but not enough to make a complete living from. I was still struggling with Fibromyalgia pain and doing TP therapy with Linda and by myself. The TP therapy was helping, but my doctor wanted to try a new drug called Prozac he had recently read about. He explained that when my body was fighting pain, my brain produced a chemical which was used by the body to deal with that pain. Excessive pain would cause the body to use more of that chemical than the brain could produce. Prozac was supposed to help my body produce more of that chemical and thus reduce the pain I was experiencing. He wrote a six month prescription for me and gave me a months supply of samples to help defray the cost of the medicine. It was fairly expensive.

He had another idea for me, too. "Since the Postal Service didn't take my word or the Myotherapist's word for the cause of your Fibromyalgia, they would believe the word of the Cleveland Clinic wouldn't they?" he said. "I am an associate doctor with them and could set up an appointment if that's OK with you. Besides, it would confirm what we already know and eliminate any further need of a diagnosis, and if they find something else which we've missed, then that's good, too." I agreed that it may be what we need to convince the Postal Service that Fibromyalgia is a legitimate condition and to convince the Workman's Compensation board to agree to pay for the medical bills from a work related condition. People are referred to the Cleveland Clinic from all over the world. It is especially known for musculo-skeletal disorders among other things. I got an appointment for late January.

I began taking Prozac just after the third week of November and continued taking it until sometime around the first of April. The experience was sort of a roller coaster ride. For the first few weeks it was like standing in line waiting with excited anticipation for what was hoped to be something good. After the first week I noticed no change whatsoever and asked the doctor what to look for. He told me that he actually didn't know what to look for since the drug was still fairly new. He did warn me of a tendency toward suicide as one of the known side effects and to discontinue taking the drug if I noticed any thoughts in that direction. With all that I had been through so far, I assured him that if I had the tendency toward suicide I would have attempted it long before now. He laughed but still warned me of that side effect.

Two more weeks went by and then three months with no noticeable changes in my body other than a light "drugged" feeling. I noticed some definite feelings of strong financial panic once or twice which I thought could have been from taking the drug, but then, a very noticeable side effect came during supper one evening. Usually, my family talked and laughed and had fun at the supper table and this night was no exception. During the fun and conversation, I told a story which was uproariously funny to everyone. The next night, the kids asked me to retell the story from the night before. I didn't know what they were talking about. I didn't remember telling a story that night. They tried to refresh my memory by telling me what they remembered of the story but it didn't help. I was blank as to what I said or did the previous evening. That scared me quite a bit causing me to wonder what else I may have said or done that I don't have memory of. I stopped taking Prozac after that incident. The entire time span of when I was taking Prozac is mostly a vague memory with only sporadic incidents and details being able to recall clearly. For a year or so after that, I still had some memory blanks and feelings of financial panic that I feel were related to taking the drug.

During that time of taking Prozac, I was called to come down to the Post Office. They didn't say why or if they did, I don't remember now. When I arrived, the postmaster introduced me to a man who was there to ask me some questions about my job and my physical problems. He told me that he was an inspector and showed me a badge from his wallet. I remember feeling glad that I was going to get to tell someone else in the Postal Service about Fibromyalgia and that job stress can cause it. At first, he listened to me, then he opened a folder and showed me a form sheet asking me if I recognized it. It was the health status form which was filled out on my first day of work at the Post Office. The one the supervisor read aloud to me while he checked off the items. I didn't recall that at the time. He pointed out the place where "no" had been checked for the item "back problems". I told him that I had always been open about my physical history and that I didn't know why I would have marked "no" on the form. I also told him that my problem was not in my back as such, but throughout the muscles in my body. He didn't seem to have much of a response to that. I know there was more conversation after that, but I only recall bits of it. The Postal Service accused me of lying about my health history after that. I did remember later that the supervisor was the one who actually filled in the blanks on that form and told them about it. He, of course, denied ever having done such a thing. I was left feeling betrayed by the system again and being wracked with muscle spasms and tension from the encounter. The union felt confident that I should fight their accusations, saying I had a good case since my problem was not in my back but in my muscles.

To some people, Prozac was like a wonder drug and helped them immensely. To others, like myself, it was a bad experience filled with confusion with no apparent gain from it.

Andrew H. Knapp - The Roses and the Oasis

Cleveland Clinic

The Cleveland Clinic appointment came quickly in the midst of the tumultuous times of taking Prozac. I recall this visit surprisingly well. I drove to Cleveland alone, stopping at every rest area to work TP's and do stretches. It's the one time where I wonder if the Prozac helped me to make the long trip tolerable or if it is just that I had been out of the work environment of the Postal Service for long enough that I was feeling the benefits of that. A good friend in Cleveland had a place for me to spend the night. In the morning I went to the clinic, registered and waited for the appointed time. A clear confirmation diagnosis of Fibromyalgia was what I hoped for from the visit. A confirmation from a place as reputable as the Cleveland Clinic was what I felt was needed to sway the Workman's Comp. board to agree that my condition was work related so the accumulated bills could be paid through that. The worry of how those bills would be paid for and where the money would come from if Workman's Comp. didn't agree to pay hung heavily over me keeping me in a state of tension. That, combined with the fears of my financial future in any workplace, made it difficult to get ahead in the TP therapy and stretching and loosening of the muscles in my body.

When I was called to come back to the examination rooms, I carried with me all the negative test results, the X-rays, CT scans and an MRI which showed nothing wrong, and the letters from the Myotherapist and my personal doctor along with the hope that this visit would be worthwhile and not an experience like the one in Indianapolis.

I had waited only a few minutes when a doctor entered the room. He looked over the packet of test results and letters I had brought. He asked me about my range of motion and where pain intensified. When I told him that I didn't have to move to have pain, he smiled and nodded. He touched a few places on my upper body. Each touch was on a Trigger Point! He knew where to find them! He said, "I don't need to check every point in your body, it is very clear to me that you have Fibromyalgia." He then asked me questions which no other doctor or institutional therapist had asked before. "Do you care about your work? Are you conscientious in what you do? Are you concerned with the feelings of others? Do you go out of your way to help others?... My voice cracked and I wept as I answered all of his questions positively. There was compassion and understanding in his eyes. He continued, "Are you satisfied with anything less than your best? Do you go out of your way to be honest in your dealings with others? Are you hurt when others are disappointed in you? Do you try to ease others burdens and troubles? Are you compassionate toward others?" I could barely answer his questions with words. I was so happy that he understood how I felt. He spoke again smiling, "The other doctors didn't believe you when their tests turned out negative. They didn't look at the person you are. In your job in the Postal Service, they didn't care about you, only the numbers you produced. I have seen this happen to caring people like you before." He then confirmed what I already knew. "I must tell you that this is not a disabling condition. It may feel like it is, but it's not. You must remove yourself from the stress causing this. If that means leaving your job, then so be it." It seemed clear to me that there was nothing in the Postal Service for me anymore, even a different job within the system would still have the same management style. I asked him about careers in the music trades, specifically piano tuning, which I had been contemplating going into. He thought piano tuning would be a good trade for a caring person to be in. He also thought that being independent without a boss or a time clock would be therapeutic for me, too. I then asked him about the TP therapy I was doing and described what Linda did and what I myself did showing him the Backnobber and how I used it. He listened and watched with interest then nodded saying, "If what you're doing causes the muscles to release their spasm, then go for it. From the look of your test results, you won't be doing your body any harm, and if it lessens the pain, I'm happy for you." He then got up to leave telling me his colleague would be in shortly.

In about ten minutes another doctor came in. He was older and spoke very little. When he finished examining me, I asked him what he found. He answered, "You have quite a case of Fibromyalgia." When I asked him what I should do about it, he simply said, "You just need a different career that's not so stressful." And that was it. I was happy and excited. The diagnosis of Fibromyalgia was confirmed! Now maybe the Workman's Comp. board would rule in my favor and pay the bills.

Massage Therapy

During the month before the memory blank incident, I noticed a sign at a beauty shop/tanning facility which read, "Massage Therapist". I stopped in to inquire what a massage therapist does, if TP therapy was part of it, etc., when, lo and behold, an old friend of mine from childhood walked out to greet me. He was the massage therapist! We were both very happy to see each other. We caught up in a few minutes and then I told him of my situation and asked my questions. Kevin knew all about Trigger Point therapy, although he called it muscle spasm release therapy. He assured me that the massage therapy he performed would help lessen the pain I was experiencing. I was thrilled! Maybe Kevin's therapy would be as effective as Suzen's Myotherapy had been. My home therapy was slow because I was so tired and fatigued much of the time that it was a struggle for me to just do the work of TP therapy with the pain and stretches it required. I needed something more at this point. Kevin found a place on his schedule for early the next day to mostly work on my neck and upper shoulders, which were in the most urgent need of work.

At Kevin's office the next morning, I went back to the massage room and undressed down to shorts and a towel. Kevin darkened the room and played peace evoking music on the stereo for the background mood. He explained to me that he was first going to loosen the outer muscles so that the individual spasms could be isolated and then released. My muscles were so tight that my own home therapy was not getting through to where the worst muscle spasms were to be able to adequately release them. I had progressed to a level where I did not have tingling or numbness in my hands and feet most of the time beginning sometime back in October or September. I also had a greater range of motion before inhibiting pain would begin.

Kevin had me lay face down on the massage table. Just the act of laying on that table with my forehead on a padded extension with my face open beneath was very relaxing. I mentioned to Kevin how comfortable the table was and that I wished my bed had an attachment for my forehead like that, too. He agreed as he applied a special massage oil and began gently but strongly to loosen the muscles in my upper back and neck area. It felt so soothing and relaxing that I asked Kevin if it would be OK if I slept while he worked. He said it would be fine and that it happens often.

With Kevin's work there was not as much intense or strong pain. When there was, I told him the level of intensity and the nerve path it followed. He would respond with something like, "Yea, I thought it would be a bad one from the size of the knot in the muscle here." He would also prepare me for the times when he knew there would be strong pain. "I have a TP isolated here, are you ready? Be sure to tell me if it gets too much for you to take. I don't want you to jump off the table." At that point it became similar to

98

the Myotherapy sessions with my grunts and moans while I concentrated on relaxing to avoid tensing the rest of my body. Kevin didn't want me to experience that level of pain. He knew there would be some pain to force the spasms to let go, but he wanted it to be done more gently. Most people were not able to concentrate on relaxing the muscles while experiencing sharp pain in them the way I did. I was used to the sharp pain from TP therapy. Most of the sensations I felt with Kevin were of the itchiness type which comes when blood circulation is returned to a muscle when a spasm is released. I must say that that first session was so soothing that I didn't stay awake for the whole hour.

Kevin gently prodded me awake when the session was finished. I hadn't felt that level of relaxation for such a long time that I couldn't re-member how long. He told me that he had made good progress in getting through the outer muscles to where he could feel the acute spasms beneath which were causing most of the pain in my body. He said, "Next time we'll begin to work some of the worst TP's, although there's still alot of loosening of the outer muscles to do. We're only just beginning to scratch the surface. You'll feel the progress each day we work the muscles." I asked about my own home TP therapy and stretches. He said, "You'll get to the acute spasms in the scapula better now. Be careful that you don't press too hard all at once or it might send you through the ceiling." We chuckled. "I have another time slot for you this Thursday at 9:30am, is that OK?" I said, "Wild horses couldn't keep me away. I haven't felt such progress since I saw the Myotherapist in Chicago."

There was a lump in my throat. I left Kevin's office that day feeling that I had found the way to get ahead of the Fibromyalgia pain in my body. I knew that once I got to the place where the major TP's were released to where they did not put pressure on the nerves or nerve paths anymore, then I would truly be able to retrain the muscles through stretching and exercise which would put **me** in control of Fibromyalgia rather than Fibromyalgia controlling me. I didn't want to do anything else other than to get above the painful condition of my body.

I was still struggling with the U.S. Postal Service and my employment status with that organization. The union told me that a job change within the system away from delivering the mail could be negotiated without much difficulty. It was the system that was killing me, though. Each time I met with the management or spoke with a union representative, the tension would grow in my shoulders and neck at first and then spread to my jaw and other parts of my body. I didn't want to deal with them, management or union, because of the physical pain it caused each time we met. I had to though. I was trying to get them to pay for my medical bills and for vocational rehabilitation, which means training for a new career to replace the job which caused the Fibromyalgia condition in my body. The Postal Service held that it was not the job that was the source of my condition, I was the source of it because of the way I handled (or rather couldn't handle) stress. "It's not the job, it's the person," they said. It was mentally draining for me to face the injustice of the situation. Trying to resolve my situation with the Postal Service was keeping me from getting above the muscle spasm condition in my body. The tension from the stress of dealing with my employer-turned-enemy was keeping me in the Fight or Flight mode and, being unable to flee from the stress, I was sitting and taking it, absorbing it into my body.

That day I left Kevin's office, I decided that somehow I had to find an end to my dealings with the Postal Service. My window of opportunity came when the Workman's Compensation board ruled in my favor to pay the accumulated medical bills for the tests and specialists visits. They even paid the Myotherapist's bill. However, they would not go so far as to agree that I needed another job to remove me from the source of the stress which caused the trouble to begin with. I finally chose to resign my position with the U.S. Postal Service. Choosing, rather, to rise above Fibromyalgia first. Fibromyalgia was the real enemy not my employers. It was a fearful thing to do, resigning from the best source of income I ever had. I was on my own now. My wife, Linda, had found a job back in the fall which offered family health insurance coverage beginning in January the next year. Things were starting to fall into place. *I noticed a thinning of the leaves in the branches above me.*

I purchased a correspondence course in Piano Tuning and Technology and began studying for a new career. I went to massage therapy sessions with Kevin two times a week for one month, then once a week for four more months. I had found a position playing church music which paid a stipend each week.

Along with the performance money, every little bit made a difference. Within three months after resigning from the Postal Service, I had gained substantially in muscle pain levels. I no longer had movement stifling pain. The overall body heaviness had diminished greatly. Kevin's therapy had worked through all of the outer muscles in my body to where he was able to release the deep TP spasms themselves. *I thanked the water for being there...then I rolled over, completely immersing myself in it's healing.*

I began to do things I hadn't done for a long time. I used the string bass at my storytelling performances again and began using movements I had curtailed from certain stories because of the stifling pain they would meet.

I tuned the piano of every friend I knew and my mother's and my own piano I tuned and re-tuned. Piano tuning came naturally to me. It felt as though I had "come home" to the trade. Having been a professional trombonist since the age of 16, my ear for music was already in place. It just needed some direction and purpose.

In August, I kicked off my piano tuning business with a booth at the 4-H Fair where I booked two tunings per day for the next three and a half months. I purchased a few ads in some local publications and came out in the phone book yellow pages in the winter edition. I was filled with excitement and enthusiasm. It felt good to be making money again in a promising new career. Most of all, it just felt good to feel good.

The pain levels in my body had gotten to a level where I even forgot about it sometimes. That hadn't happened in so long I couldn't remember when. Linda and the kids were happy to have papa back. I could play and run and have fun again. I had visions of living a carefree life someday. Oh, how I wanted that freedom. But, every day I gave myself to the discipline of my stretching and exercises routine. Every time I felt TP pain I used the Backnobber or a knuckle or my bicycle seat or the top of the stair rail to allay the muscle spasms. I was working at getting ahead of and above Fibromyalgia. I was really doing it!

Over the following months of feeling less and less pain in my body, I developed an attitude of trying anything. Through my education along the path of diagnosing Fibromyalgia and the therapy journey, as I stated earlier, I learned that the pain from Fibromyalgia muscle spasms is not "real" as in other ailments. The spasms place pressure on nerves as they pass through the muscles and the pressure is interpreted by the brain as pain in other parts of the body away from where the source of the pressure really is. With that knowledge of the "false pain" from Fibromyalgia, my attitude changed to an "I can do anything I want to do, if it causes pain then I'll handle it when it comes, if it doesn't, then good. I won't let the fear of causing pain keep me from living." A level of arrogance came with that attitude. It wasn't an entirely bad thing, though. I found that I was working hard at everything I did. From working to exercising to stretching to playing. It was as if life

103

had been given back to me and I wasn't going to miss any of it because of the fear of pain.

I made it through the thorns.

—————

The Window in the Corridor
a story

I found myself in a long, dimly lit corridor of some kind moving at a brisk pace following in a line of people to where I did not know.

I watched the sweat run down in patterns on the person's back in front of me.

We all seemed to be jogging along in unison with the person's step ahead of us apparently to avoid tangling our feet and falling or slowing down the progress of the line.

In the center of the corridor, although I couldn't actually see them in the dim light, were large, gruff-voiced people spaced at intervals along the way who each held a whip in one hand and a very loud police-type whistle in the other.

They yelled commands as the line proceeded along.

"Stay in line!"
"Don't slow down!"
"Keep your eyes straight ahead!"
"No looking around!"

The whip would lash out at anyone who would not conform to the flow of the line.

A whistle would blow just before each lash and snap of a whip.

Each whistle and snap echoed far down the corridor blending with the yelling and the shuffling and padding of feet to create an oppressive din.

Dust hung in the air causing me to choke and cough often.

My mind was blank.

I had no thoughts or memories.

I only knew that I had to stay in line.

The all important line.

I didn't know why I was in this line or what the purpose of the line was.

I was just there.

Obediently and fearfully there.

Suddenly, above the din in the corridor, a loud alarm sounded.

The line abruptly stopped, doors, unnoticed along the walls before, opened to brightly lit rooms and commands were shouted accompanied by whistles and whip cracks ordering everyone into the rooms.

I squinted in the bright light.

Each person was given tasks to perform while in the room.

What the tasks were is only a vague memory now.

The tasks in the room came almost as a relief from the monotony of the corridor.

Time passed quickly while we were occupied with the tasks.

After an unknown span of time, another alarm sounded, the doors of the rooms opened and everyone was ordered into the corridor again to resume following the line.

I felt numb and empty.

I made no sound nor did I resist as I fell into place in the line.

As I moved along with the flow of the line, thoughtlessly watching the back of the person in front of me, time lost what little meaning it had as one step followed another in the dust and roar of the corridor.

I looked up for no apparent reason.

When I did, I saw a window just out of reach further ahead down the corridor.

A glimmer of something in my memory came back.

What was it?

I could see blue sky through the window, I caught a whiff of a freshness in the stifling air of the corridor.

Blue sky?

Fresh air?

A whistle blew followed by a whip lash and crack aimed at me.

"Keep your head down and your eyes forward!"

"No looking around!"

Another moment later the alarm sounded, the doors opened and everyone filed into the rooms again.

I had difficulty doing the tasks this time.

The window, along with a distant memory of something pleasant, burned in my thoughts.

There was something about the sky...I felt a stirring deep inside...a real memory.

I had to see the sky again!

The alarm sounded at its unknown time, the doors opened, everyone filed into the corridor to resume following the line again,...except me.

The moment I entered the corridor, I made a dash for the window.

I leaped and grabbed the windowsill.

The sky was out there!

Whistles and whip cracks sounded behind and below me.

They yelled at me to come down and tried to catch my feet, but I pulled myself up and through the window.

I tumbled out onto a soft grassy meadow, rolled down a hill, and just sat there in a daze.

No one pursued me.

I was out.

All was quiet and calm.

Peace filled me.

I gazed into the sky.

The air was fresh and clean and I breathed deeply of it.

I looked out over the countryside and saw grass, flowers, insects, birds, trees, hills and mountains in the distance.

I sat there for hours, or was it days, breathing in the ecstasy of the moment.

I stood up finally, and began wandering.

I had no destination.

I was filled with wonder and awe at the peace and beauty that surrounded me.

The sky.

The open sky above me.

It felt good to be free.

I was not conscious of time.

I wandered for countless hours enjoying the moments.

Somewhere among the wanderings, I found myself on a path.

It was a faint, barely recognizable, small path at first, but as I followed it, it became more defined.

It felt good to be on a path.

I followed the path.

It led me to a high place where I could see far ahead and down the path.

I saw another person walking on the path far ahead of me.

It felt good to see another person, though I did not try to catch up.

The path descended into a valley and curved around a hill.

There, another path joined the path I followed.

I looked far up that path and saw another person following it down toward me.

I did not wait but continued following the path.

After the first adjoining path, I noticed that at each bend in my path, another path came to join it, though it seemed odd that no path crossed it.

Someone was following each path.

I began waving to the people in the distance following their paths leading into mine.

They waved back.

I thought how good it felt to greet someone and I could sense they were glad to greet me, too.

I could see other people on the path with me now.

Some ahead of me and others behind.

The sun shone down warm and a gentle breeze blew soft on my body.

Beautiful clouds came and washed me, the others, and the land around with gentle rain.

Everything felt good.

No one spoke.

But one day the sun shone strong and hot with no wind.

Someone broke the silence and spoke.

"It's too hot out here."

No one had thought that way before.

All things were peacefully accepted as they came.

I noticed that the path was becoming smoother and wider with many more people following the path.

At every curve another path still joined the main path with someone following each one.

It began to rain again.

Someone further ahead spoke.

"We need to get out of this rain."

Many others around me agreed.

I heard a grumbling and murmuring from most of the others on the path.

I looked ahead and could see groups of people building a roof over the path.

The path led under the roof.

It felt good to be under the roof out of the rain and the hot sun.

Everyone felt relieved.

A strong wind began to blow.

At first, the wind felt good, but then someone spoke.

"The wind is too strong."

More grumbling and murmuring echoed under the roof of the path.

Then I heard hammering ahead and saw groups of people building walls along the path to shield everyone from the wind.

It felt good, at first, to be out of the wind, but it became dark inside the roof and walls of the path.

I noticed incandescent lights hanging from the rafters as I followed along.

The path curved and went downhill, then leveled out.

I heard a faint roaring sound in the distance.

It grew gradually louder with each step.

With no rain or wind, the dust rose in clouds as we followed the path.

It became difficult to breathe without choking and coughing.

The roaring sound grew louder and closer.

I suddenly recognized the sound!

Whistles and whip lashes and cracks.

Yelling and shouting of commands.

I looked up, noticing a window going by...

I didn't hesitate.

Before anyone could force me to stay in line, I leaped for the window, held onto the sill and pulled myself out...

to freedom.

---

*See page 135, #19b, for explanation of story.

The Continuing Story

Over the months and years after rising above Fibromyalgia control of my body, I performed a daily stretching and exercise routine. Every morning upon getting out of bed, I would begin with full arm circles, both forward and backward. The same as a baseball pitcher warms up only with both arms together. I did about ten rotations in each direction. Following this, while still standing, I would place both hands behind my neck, as if to do sit-ups, held my elbows as far back as possible pulling my shoulders back and, while holding the shoulders back, extended my arms directly overhead and then slowly made an outward circle coming around to cross in front of my body and up to the top of the circle, then bringing the hands to the back of the neck to begin again. I did ten of these also. While still standing, I did the neck/scapula stretch. Turning my head to about a 45 degree angle to one side, I would tilt my head down using my chin as a pointer toward the floor and hold for a 30 second count, repeating on the other side. This was followed by straight forward and back head nods, side to side head tilts, and side to side rotations. These were done for two slow repetitions of ten seconds on each side. After this, I did a full upper body twist rotation with my head turning to look over my shoulder on each side and holding my arms in a bent-elbow jogging position. I kept my eyes open to prevent dizziness. I usually did about 20 repetitions back and forth. I then got down on the floor to stretch the lower back and gluteus (buttocks). While lying flat on my back, I would raise my knees up and pull them to my chest with my hands, holding for at least 30 seconds. (If you are going to start using these exercises now, there is one gluteus (buttock) stretch which I did not know of until about three years later, which helps immensely. After doing the knees to the chest stretch, keep one knee held to the chest while straightening the other. Grasp the toes of the leg held up with the other hand and gently pull them down toward the opposite side of the body and hold for 30 seconds. For example, the right knee is held with the right hand and the right toes are grasped with the left hand and pulled toward the left side of the body. You should feel the stretch deep within the gluteus muscle. Repeat with the other leg. This exercise is extremely important in preventing sciatic nerve problems and associated leg pain.) I then did repetitions of 30 knee to chest raises, touching my elbows to my knees each time with my hands behind my neck, eventually working up to 80 or 100, for abdominal muscle exercise. A strong abdomen can prevent backaches. From this position, I would roll over to do the "camel and cat" back stretch. This entails first getting on hands and knees, then slowly lifting the head up as comfortably high as possible while arching the back by pushing the abdomen down, then slowly lowering the head down to stretch the back in the opposite direction as comfortably far as possible. Do this for at least 15 seconds for each direction. Next, I would sit on the floor and do some leg stretches, like those done in track and field warm ups. With legs spread to a 90 degree angle with toes pointed up, I reached as far as possible, without straining, toward one foot, just enough to feel a stretch, and hold for at least 20 seconds. Repeat with the other foot. After this, I stood to do the curtsy toe stretch. I would place the top of the toes of one foot behind the other foot and bend the knee of the supporting leg, slightly stretching the shin and top of the foot of the back leg for a 20 second count or more, then repeating with the other foot. I was then ready for the day. I always carried my trusty Backnobber with me to stop muscle spasms which would come now and then throughout the day. I recognized these as generally localized pain in one muscle or another. There usually wasn't referred pain until I used the Backnobber on the spasm to release it. I was very persistent in doing my stretching and exercises every day. My freedom of movement and freedom from stifling pain depended on it.

As my physical state became easier and easier to maintain, however, there were days when I skipped exercising or omitted some stretches out of convenience or simply laziness. I think some of it may have come from a "cocky" arrogance or complacence I developed along the way. Sort of like "It won't happen to me again".

Relapse and Recovery

Business was OK but could have been better. During the months of mid-winter, calls for piano tunings usually slowed down causing us to seek new ways to get more customers. In the spring of 1995, Linda heard of a piano tuner who was moving out of the area and selling his business of regular customers. I contacted him and worked out a deal where I purchased his business.

Wow! did I ever shift gears to step into that! I began tuning three and four pianos a day. Before that I usually tuned two a day. I came home at the end of each day exhausted but excited that business was so good. However, the pressure to tune all those pianos and the exhaustion began to cut into my daily exercise time more than before. Even prior to the purchase of the other piano business, I had been lax in some of the exercises. Also during this time of early summer, there were visits from a few out of town friends which lasted for several days at a time over a span of about three weeks. The way I love good conversation, this caused me to stay up later on those nights which cut into my sleep time. Lost sleep is nearly impossible to make up for with a full business schedule to keep. I began to skip exercises altogether on days when I had early morning tunings or when I didn't get enough sleep the night before, sometimes skipping two or three days at a time.

117

In July of 1995, the toll of being lax in my stretching and exercises and the stress of keeping up with the new business and the intervals of lost sleep, caught up with my body. I had noticed some of the early pain signs in my legs and gluteus before this, but chose to ignore it with the "it won't happen again" attitude. I awoke one morning with sharp nerve pain zinging down my right leg all the way to my toes. The muscles in the lumbar vertebrae region of my lower back and gluteus had gone into deep spasm putting pressure on the sciatic nerve as it passed through them. I could barely get out of bed, the pain was so strong and sharp. I immediately began trying to release the Trigger Points in that area of my muscles using the top of the stair rail and the Backnobber. The pain was so intense that the old familiar pain-panic-desperation nearly set in. I concentrated on controlling my body's reactions to the sharp, gripping pain.

After working the muscles for 10 to 15 minutes, I was able to calm the spasms enough to get dressed. The movement of walking around in the house seemed to lessen the intensity of the pain down my leg. I called my doctor to ask if there were any non-drowsy medications I could take and to see if there was room for an appointment that day. There were two pianos to tune at a church on the schedule located only five miles away. I was able to tune the first piano by intermittently tuning for 5 or 6 minutes, getting up and working TP's when the spasms increased with sharp pain shooting down my leg, doing some gluteus stretches, walking around a little, then tuning more of the piano again. It took at least

118

an hour longer to tune that piano that day. I decided to tune the other piano on another day after I felt better again. I went home to work TP's, stretch and try to catch up on some rest. My previous nights sleep had not been very restful. The doctor's office squeezed me in for an afternoon appointment where I was given a prescription for Naproxin and Parafon Forte. These were supposedly the least drowsiness inducing medications for pain available. I told my doctor what I was doing to try to stop the muscle spasms with TP therapy and stretching exercises. He acknowledged that, by now, I probably knew more about muscle spasm therapy and what to do about it than most conventional doctors and physical therapists. By the evening I had the sharp sciatic leg pains fairly under control, or so I thought. Linda was glad to hear that I was able to control it, but she was obviously worried.

The next morning began earlier than the previous morning with more of the sharp, intense sciatic pain shooting down my leg again. I did the same as before working the TP's until I felt I had gained some headway against the pain. This day, though, I had three tunings scheduled in a town located 40 minutes from home. I had my Backnobber with me, which I used while driving, but the muscle spasms had grown too much for me to handle this time while sitting in a driving position for that length of time. I was forced to panic stop several times along the highway to jump out of the van so I could move and stretch my leg due to the intensity of the pain. When I finally arrived at the house of my first appointment, I couldn't sit down long enough to set up the piano for tuning. The piano was a short upright, so I tried to kneel while installing the mutes. The pain kept coming no matter what position I was in. I realized that I was not going to tune any pianos that day, so I apologized to the woman whose house I was in and explained some of my predicament. She understood and empathized with me immediately saying that whenever I could get her back on the schedule would be fine as long as I got the pain taken care of first.

I knew what it felt like to have intense sciatic pain. The memory of the first time, from back in 1982, when it affected my left leg, came back very clearly in my mind. It was like meeting an old enemy who had defeated me once before, coming back to beat me down again. Only this time, I didn't have the fear of the unknown to hinder me. I did have the knowledge and the determination to deal with it, though.

It seemed to take forever to get home from that "40 minute" drive. It took more than twice as long. Every time I put my foot on the accelerator and held my leg in the driving position for more than a few minutes, the muscles in the lower back and gluteus would go into severe spasms sending intense, sharp pain down my leg. I was only able to drive a few blocks before having to stop and get out of the van to shift position and to move. The movement helped but the Backnobber was not enough to stop the spasms. As before, it was like throwing a rock into a raging torrent in an attempt to control the flow. It worked wonderfully well on the smaller muscle spasms when only part of a muscle was giving problems, but this was too much for it all at once to manage. I didn't even think about going to a hospital emergency room. I knew that an emergency room doctor wouldn't be able to do anything, except to sedate me, to stop the pain. I knew I needed concentrated TP therapy, stretches and rest. I knew what to do, it was getting home to do it that was my problem at that moment.

I finally got to the highway, which was a four lane interstate type road. I was glad to have plenty of room to stop and get out. After a few stops, it occurred to me to get the van up to speed, set the speed control and move my right leg to any position that was semi pain free and see how long I could go like that. The first try I lasted about five minutes before spasms forced me off the road. The second try lasted more than ten minutes because I had found the best position, which provoked the least amount of muscle spasms, during the first try. Eventually, I had to exit the highway and drive five miles the normal way to get home. I decided to drive the last part using my left foot on the gas and brake while holding my right leg in a comfortable position. This worked very well with only a few times when my left foot hit the brake too hard. I was exhausted when I finally got home.

Linda knew what the trouble was as soon as she saw me. I asked her to work the TP's in the gluteus muscles, the lower back and the back of the thighs. I got onto the table in the basement and Linda worked TP's using her elbows mostly. I was so glad that she knew what to do and could do it effectively. After she finished and I did some stretches, all I wanted to do was to lay down and sleep. But first, I had to call my customers who were scheduled for that day and the rest of the week to ask them to re-schedule a time later on in the month and I apologized for any inconvenience this caused them. I then laid down on the couch, got my leg to a comfortable position and fell asleep...for about 20 minutes. Muscle spasms and sciatic pain jolted me awake. I jumped up, walked around the room a little, then went upstairs to work TP's in those muscles using the top of the stair rail. While using the top of the stair rail, I could put most of my body weight into the pressure on the TP's in the large gluteus muscles and also in the lower splenius muscles in the lower back and the muscles in the back of the thighs. I found that I could put the pressure closer to the exact spot in the muscle when I did it myself using the stair rail. This settled the biggest spasms for a while. I stretched the muscles as best I could, fell onto the bed, curled into the most comfortable position, which was almost fetal position, and fell asleep for nearly an hour this time.

Upon waking, I went downstairs and walked around in the house until time for supper. I was unable to stand still or sit still for more than a minute or two. While standing, I found that shaking my leg felt better than not moving it. I paced around the house. Sometimes back and forth, sometimes standing and shaking my leg, sometimes pacing and shaking my leg as I paced. At supper, I couldn't sit long enough to eat very much before needing to get up and pace around the room. I was sort of eating on the run. Everyone felt bad for me. They were helpless spectators watching as I wandered around in pain.

After supper, we all went for a walk. While walking, the pain was much less intense than while stationary. We walked for quite a while. An hour or more. I didn't want to stop walking since the pain was so much more tolerable when doing so, but everyone else had walked enough. I resumed the pacing and shaking not long after getting home and it went on that way until time for bed.

Bed, Ha! I tried sleeping but the pain kept waking me up. I tossed and turned for a long time without finding a lasting comfortable position. I finally went downstairs to try sleeping in the easy chair in order to give Linda some peaceful sleep without me tossing and turning and moaning and groaning right beside her. It was about 1:00am.

Between 3:30 and 4:00am, after two and a half hours of fitful sleep with no real rest, I began hearing the birds singing outside before dawn. I could see the sky getting lighter in the east. I remembered, then, something I had read in my Fibromyalgia research years earlier. It had to do with musculo-skeletal functioning with regards to aerobic exercise. I think it was in the book on Osteopathic medicine and in the Australian research on Repetitive Stress Syndrome.

The facts are these: When the body is engaged in aerobic exercise, such as running, swimming, cross-country skiing, bicycling, paddling, rowing, etc., the bones in the spine are lifted slightly apart by the muscles of the body, thereby taking pressure off the discs between the vertebrae, enhancing the cushioning effect of the discs when at rest and at other times. Also, when the muscles are engaged in aerobic exercise, the heat generated by the body eases the tensions of muscle spasms. This fact also pointed me to the fact that higher body heat brings about an acid reaction in the blood causing the blood to flow better allowing it to reach into the constricted capillaries within a muscle spasm and thus lessen the muscle spasm.

When those facts came together in my mind, I went upstairs, put on my gym shorts and running shoes, told Linda what facts had just hit my mind and that I was going out to do some running. I had nothing to lose except the pain. I ran at least four miles that morning, stopping once in a while to do some stretches, talk to God and lose myself in the beauty of the unfolding day. I was out for more than an hour.

By the time I got home I felt better. Not just for a few minutes, but better! When I worked the TP's in the lower back, buttocks, and thigh muscles, it was much more effective and longer lasting. I was able to reach the deep muscle spasms because the outer muscles had relaxed from the heat of the exercise activity. Throughout the rest of that day, I worked TP's and stretched. When I slept during the day, I was able to sleep for over two hours comfortably. That night I slept for nearly five hours. When I awoke with the birds again, I worked TP's, did stretches and some abdominal exercises, and went out and ran again. It was better than the first day of running. I was still in the woods, but the underbrush was thinning ahead of me.

During this time, I was taking the prescription pain killers and muscle relaxants, too. I had taken three doses of those medications by the time I started running, which could make just about the level of being able to help in my body. As with most prescription pill medications, it takes a few doses for there to be enough of the substance in the body's system to have positive effect. Some require several days of taking the medicine for there to be enough in the system to begin having an effect. I don't know if there was enough in my body's system or not. All I knew at the time was that I was getting better through the running aerobic exercise I was doing. I still took the medicines twice each day as the doctor prescribed, but I am sure it was the running that did the most to break through the muscles. I think the aerobics loosened the outer muscles in sort of the same way as the massage therapy did to be able to penetrate to the inner, deep Trigger Point muscle spasms which cause the pressure on the nerves.

By the third morning of running, the major muscle spasms causing the sciatic pain in my leg had subsided down to levels which were easily manageable. I was **happy!** I felt as though I had wrestled with a formidable foe and won! I had won the battle with Fibromyalgia! Not the war, that will last a lifetime. Now that I knew what to do and how to recognize it and fight it, I could keep the enemy on the run. Back in 1982 when Fibromyalgia first showed it's ugly head in the form of sciatic pain in my left leg, I lost eight weeks of work because of it. This time in 1995, I lost only five days of work. I knew what it was this time! I knew what to do! I was not paralyzed by fear and the unknown as was the case the first time. I acted with confidence armed with knowledge.

Since that time to the present, **I** have been in control of the Fibromyalgia in my body.

Epilogue

Ever since that time, I work hard at getting to bed on time to allow for eight, no less than seven, hours of sleep. I make sure to balance my diet, drink plenty of fluids, get enough fiber, eat much less meat and, above all, keep a positive attitude about life. I do aerobic exercise, on a routine, three times a week. I get up early after my seven or eight hours of sleep, do stretches, abdominal exercises and some push-ups to balance the workout to include most of the body, and then go out and run for no less than 20 minutes. Not like running a race, just a steady jog. Enough to produce a sweat and then sustain that pace for 20 minutes or more. The reason for no less than 20 minutes is that during aerobic exercise the cardiovascular system reaps it's greatest benefits for the body after about 18 or 20 minutes of continual movement. If you're going to go running to help remove muscle spasms, then it makes good sense to run for a minimum of 20 minutes to benefit the heart as well as the muscles. It's like getting two for the price of one. Be sure to consult with your doctor before you go running for the first time, especially if you have never done it before, just in case there is something other than muscle spasms you need to work on.

There are two more things I need to tell you about running. The first is setting a pace. Most people don't think about breathing when they run or exercise, they just do it. Over the years, I have learned that when a person is jogging, breathing usually is on an even numbered pattern, two steps inhale two steps exhale. Also, the first step on each inhale and the first step on each exhale strikes the ground harder than the second. With that in mind, if you begin your jogging breath on your right foot, it will be striking the ground harder than the left during the entire time you are jogging. I don't know where I learned it, but whenever I jog, I use an odd numbered pattern to balance out the strike foot to every other foot with each inhale. For example, two steps inhale three steps exhale, makes the strike foot rotate from the right foot on one inhale to the left foot on the next inhale, thus balancing the body. It takes some concentration at first, but after a while it becomes a habit. Exhaling more than inhaling has another benefit in that more of the body's wastes are removed to provide for a more efficient use of the oxygen that is inhaled. Those with asthma will benefit from the greater amount of exhale, since the asthmatic lungs tend to constrict the air passages preventing complete exhales. Behind all of this is that **you** are in control of your body and conscious of everything that goes on inside of it.

As you work yourself through Fibromyalgia pain and TP therapy, you will eventually be able to recognize muscle pain and differentiate between that pain and other sources of pain in your body. It is of the utmost importance to be able to recognize the sensations which lead up to the muscle spasm/pain scenario. Notice when you are tensing your shoulders and holding them forward or clenching your teeth or holding your eyebrows down, etc. Learn to relax as soon as you recognize you are holding tension. Lower your shoulders, lift your head, relax your face and jaw or whatever part of your body you are tensing. When pains such as deep pin pricks or an inner pinching or gripping sensation of a certain area or muscle are noticed, action must be taken to remove the spasm as soon as possible and not ignored, to prevent Fibromyalgia pain from following it's former course in the body, leading to an inhibition of movement and the limiting of freedom for the individual. The temptation is to yield to the fatigue, (it is very tiring to fight pain, work out muscle spasms and do stretching and exercises) and convince yourself that more sleep and rest will be what the body needs to get rid of it's spasms. The opposite, however, is true. When your body's muscles are in the spasms of Fibromyalgia, rest alone will not help. Muscles that are in spasm and holding onto it, will not let go unless forced to through massage and TP therapy followed by stretching and retraining of those muscles.

Your middle name needs to become Determination. You must resolve to rise above and take control of Fibromyalgia and refuse to be a captive of your own body. Think positively. Take the time to read and study. Arm yourself with knowledge, then apply that knowledge with confidence.

You can do it. The future can be good. It's all up to you.

Andrew H. Knapp - The Roses and the Oasis

———

Appendixes:

Some bits and pieces which may or
may not be in the book
(if they already are, then good)

1.   The word Fibromyalgia means, fibrous
tissue pain. Officially, it is titled a syndrome, which
is a collection of symptoms attributed to one
condition. Myofascial Pain Syndrome is a similar
condition. When I mention Fibromyalgia in the book,
I also mean Myofascial Pain Syndrome.

2.   The pain can range from a constant
deep, dull pain, to sharp cramping pain, to sharp nerve
pain, to tingling in the fingers and toes, to numbness
in various places, especially the feet and hands, to
always feeling cold, to constant fatigue with a heavy,
weighted down feeling, to depression, to the pain of
being misunderstood, of feeling alone, the pain which
comes from the fear of maybe never living without
pain, and the fear of the unknown.

3.   Muscle tissues are not destroyed by
Fibromyalgia, they are just filled with pain from
spasms which come from stress. The muscles will
lose strength from lack of use, but not from the
condition of Fibromyalgia itself.

4.   Caring, Sensitive, conscientious people
are the most likely candidates to develop the

circumstances for this condition to occur. Learn to say no when asked to volunteer or do anything that puts a strain on your schedule. Find your level of how much is too much and be stern about staying below it. There is always someone else who can help, too. You can't do everything. Your body is telling you that you shouldn't. Listen to your body.

5.   The healing of Fibromyalgia is a way of life, not an instant cure.

6.   When you find that certain movements bring on more pain, don't let that limit yourself. Set that as a goal to find which muscles are causing the pain and work out the TP's. All there is to lose is the pain and freedom is the gain.

7.   Learn the names of the muscles of the body and the nerve paths which travel through them.

8.   I used to have the sniffles and sneezes often from what I thought were "catching a chill" or some allergy, often not knowing where they came from. I also used to be very allergic to various things. I believe that the reduction of stress in my life has greatly reduced my susceptibility to getting the sniffles and sneezes.

9.   Be aware of your feelings and emotions as to how they affect your whole person.

10.   Find a trusted partner, preferably a spouse, to learn massage and Trigger Point therapy to

perform on you. Someone you can be completely relaxed with.

11.   Meditation is a good way to remove stress and relax the body and mind. I recommend the meditation formula from the book "Awakening Spirits" by Tom Brown, Jr.

12.   Find your best and easiest way to release stress in your life. Once you find it, put it into practice.

13.   Sometime in the midst of struggling with Fibromyalgia, I stopped wearing contact lenses because my eyes felt irritated all the time for no apparent reason while wearing them. From talking with others with Fibromyalgia, it seems that there is less tear production in people with this condition. In my own observation on it, however, it appears that dehydration in varying levels is common among people who are depressed. So if you are noticing more eye irritation for no apparent reason, compensate by drinking more fluids, whether you feel thirsty or not. It may even help on the muscular and cellular level to have enough fluids for basic bodily functions and possibly prevent stress from settling in the muscles.

14.   The healing of Fibromyalgia encompasses the entire person, not just the physical body.

15.   In D.C. Jarvis' book, "Folk Medicine", there are many discussions on body chemistry and how to keep one's body in the proper balance. Most of it has to do with diet and racial make-up. It is quite simple and natural. I highly recommend reading this book. In fact, I say, please read this book.

16.   Where to find the Backnobber:
The Pressure Positive Co.
128 Oberholtzer Road
Gilbertsville, PA 19525
1-610-754-6204
www.pressurepositive.com

17.   "The Roses and the Oasis" story came to me in the form of a vision during a prayer meeting in the Log Chapel at the University of Notre Dame, Notre Dame, IN.

18.   "The Window in the Corridor" story came as a dream sometime in the early 1980's. I should have listened to what it was trying to say to me back then.

19.   On the two stories, "The Roses and the Oasis" and "The Window in the Corridor", I need to mention something as to how to put their meanings to use. Stories are living things in a sense. Keep in mind that they change in their meaning and depth for each individual and remain in the memory for new understanding to sprout at other needed moments in life. The following are my own interpretations of the stories.

19a.   In the "Roses and the Oasis" story, the path in the desert represents the feeling of being the only person who feels the way you do. That you feel that you are alone in your situation. The smell of the roses represents the discovery or rumor of a possible solution to your situation. The rose thicket represents what appears, at first, to be a very pleasant answer to your problems, but, after closer examination, reveals the struggle it can take to obtain a solution to your situation.   The sound of water beyond the thicket represents a hoped for or promised solution. The path around the rose thicket represents the desire to find an easy or instant solution to any difficult situation. Sitting on the path filled with despair after circling the thicket without finding an easy way in represents the realization that the solution will require work, pain and perseverance to accomplish. The thorns represent the pain required in order to experience the healing. There are some situations in life which must be struggled through painfully in order to gain the healing at the end. The disbelief at suddenly being through the thorns represents the idea that the impossible has been accomplished. Yes, you have arrived. The thankfulness represents the appreciation of the value of what has been accomplished. Come, enjoy the fruit of your labor.

19b.   The "Window in the Corridor" story represents being stuck in a job, a routine, or a situation in which you have no control of your life. The thoughtless following along the path represents any one of us who is in a mundane or captive or abusive situation who hasn't thought about what it all means or doesn't know any difference. The window represents a possibility of something better or different. The wandering in the fields represents having something good but not knowing what to do with it. The discovery of a faint path represents the ease of falling into the old familiar pattern of the past and it's sense of security. The other paths leading to the one path represents the similar situation of each person following their own path in life and that we are not alone in seeking to follow what we know. The following along with the others on the path during the complaining about the rain, the sun and the wind represents how we often follow the desire of the crowd without thinking about what we, individually, would do. Recognizing the sounds of the former corridor represents our realization of the circle we have travelled and the repetition of our entrapment we foresee. We leap for the window we see ahead, pull ourselves out and, hopefully, use the wisdom we have gained from the experience to prevent it from happening again.

STRESS:
How do we manage it?
What happens when we can't?

Each of us has ways, or styles, to handle or manage stress in our own individual bodies. One way of saying it is, "Where do we put our stress?" "How do we handle it?" "How do we release it?"

It is very common to see people arguing and yelling and shouting at each other. We see it nearly every time we turn on the TV or watch a movie drama. Arguing, or blowing up, and yelling and shouting is a way for some people to vent the frustrations and stresses of their every day world. Much energy is expelled by screaming and shouting. It could almost be considered a form of exercise, when expressed in a positive way, and I do, in fact, believe it to be just that, a form of exercise. It is said that a good hearty laugh every day expels sickness and improves the health. It takes a good amount of energy to laugh. Hopefully, you have had the experience of laughing so hard that your cheeks hurt and your side aches. That expulsion of energy in the form of laughter exercise removes much of the stress accumulated each day. Those of us who yell and shout and blow up to vent our stress need to find laughter instead of argument as our release.

There is another audible form of release of this pent up stress which is called the "Primal Scream". You simply get into your car by yourself (or maybe alone on the elevator between floors) with the windows closed, driving or stationary, and let loose with a blood-curdling scream from deep down in the depths of your being. All the way down to your toes, so to say. If you can do this, you will find a release that maybe you have never experienced before. Try it. It works to get rid of some stress build up.

I do a Primal Scream very often, usually in the truck after finishing with the last appointment of the day on the way home. Most of my life, I can remember being able to do this. However, I recall that, after Fibromyalgia began in my body, and after struggling through it toward recovery and the management of it, I had not done Primal Screams for many months before the onset and during the recovery therapy time until I began to see the light at the end of the tunnel. Until I began to feel relief from some of the muscle pain. I think those renewed Primal Screams were screams of joy more than screams of release, but I began doing Primal Screams again and my family noticed. They told me how good it was to hear me "holler" like that again. They said it was like happiness had returned to me. By the way, those who have the closest relationships with you should be allowed to hear your Primal Scream once in a while, if possible, especially if they are screams of joy.

Many people physically release their stress. Regretfully, frustration and anger build up from work environments and spill out at totally unrelated times. Domestic violence, I feel, often times is a result of pent up stresses which are not released at the source of the stress, namely, the workplace, where a job could be lost as the result of a stress related outburst. The internalized stress comes out, for example, when a child spills a glass of milk, resulting in a battered or verbally abused child, or, when anything goes wrong at home, a fault is violently, physically and/or verbally placed on a spouse or child who just happens to be there to receive it. The ones who are most dear and close become the recipients of the physical stress release. Domestic violent stress releases, I believe, can also be the result of a subconscious blaming of the underlying source of the reason for working at all. The responsibilities of having a spouse, children and a home force us to find ways to provide a monetary income to support these domestic needs. Everyone hears of those fellow employees who do not enjoy their work or are not working in a career field they are educated in or would not be doing this if they had not gotten married or did not have children. These frustrated workers often place blame on their responsibilities, their spouse and children, for their forced labor situations and violently release their pent up stresses where the subconscious dictates. This means physical as well as verbal releases.

Fortunately, physical stress releases are dispersed in sports activities, as well. From the spectator to the participant, sports activities and contests are excellent places to release stress. Participants physically and verbally release stress, cheerleaders physically and verbally release stress, and spectators, mostly verbally and some physically, release stress, all through the excitement and festivity of a sporting event. Even if you don't have any personal connections to anyone on either side of a sports contest, such as basketball, baseball, soccer, football, volleyball, tennis or some other sporting event, a stress release is reason enough to go and give a Primal Scream with the cheerleaders or shout and holler exuberantly when your team of choice scores a goal. No one has to know it is your excuse to release your pent up stress. Besides, that's what everyone else there is doing whether they know it or not. Go to an organized sporting event in your town or neighborhood the next time you hear of one, it will do you good. Be free. Let yourself go.

Those of you who have the gift of music and can play a musical instrument have an excellent way to release stress built right in. Coming home from a difficult day at work, head straight for the piano or the music room, pick out the appropriate music for the level of stress you need to release, and play. It could be anything from Rochmaninov to Mozart to Gershwin to Chopsticks to Heart and Soul, anything you can play. Much energy is expended through the act of performing music, regardless of the instrument being played. All musical instruments require a certain amount of manual dexterity and concentration to be able to play them. Blast out your stress on a trombone, trumpet, French horn or other brass instrument. Race yourself while playing scales on a flute, clarinet, saxophone, oboe or other woodwind instrument. Tune up your guitar, banjo or mandolin and do some pickin' and strummin'. Rosin up the bow and get out your violin, viola, cello or bass and make music. Play drum rolls and rim shots, turn on the stereo and accompany your favorite songs while playing the drum set, congas, bongos or countless other percussion instruments. Your family and friends may run and hide during the process, but they will appreciate **you** better afterward.

A side note to professional instrumentalists, clerical and assembly workers, etc.: An affliction known as Repetitive Stress Syndrome is a problem which can affect musicians and other workers in the same way Tennis Elbow affects tennis players. It is a concentrated form of Fibromyalgia and can be treated and managed in much the same way. I myself am a professional instrumentalist. During the time when Fibromyalgia was developing in my body through the stress build up from my regular day job, there were times when I could not play certain instruments, especially the string bass, because of the great pain I experienced in my hands, arms, shoulders and neck. Through my recovery and education in therapy techniques and stress management, I am no longer inhibited from any musical performances. I keep a constant vigil to stay ahead of any muscle spasms and eliminate them as soon as they become evident.

You can learn this, too.

If you are not an instrumentalist, music is still a good stress release for you. Dancing to your favorite music is wonderful for the movement of body and spirit. Even if there is no one to dance with, make the effort to let the music move you. Sing along as you dance. If you can't sing then make a joyful noise. Singing is similar to a Primal Scream. The scream is just controlled when we sing. Don't worry what people will think. It is your stress release that this is all about. Besides, your carefree attitude will become contagious and they will be more free to express themselves, too. Dancing and singing combined becomes an excellent form of exercise. We've heard it all before, but here it is again. Those of us who can't or don't run for exercise can dance and sing to attain the same level of release for our pent up stress. Sometimes just being in the audience during a concert, symphony, or play affects the emotions and moves the heart enough for stress to be released while passively enjoying the show.

I am certain that I have not mentioned all the ways which people use to release their pent up stress. We are all unique in our styles of living. Look around and experiment with different ways to release stress. You will find what works the best for you. Whatever the form of release, it is extremely important to find a way for you to release your pent up stress and not hold it in for it to develop into trouble in one form or another later.

Unfortunately, there are many of us, both female and male, who simply cannot release our stress build up each day. In stressful situations, there are three choices we are each faced with. They are: fight, flight, or sit and take it. Either we resist stress and fight it, we realize stress and run from it or detach ourselves mentally to avoid it, or we have stress placed on us and we do nothing except quietly absorb it without resistance. We are too nice to let anyone be bothered or inconvenienced because of us. We can't say no even when our schedules are full. We will do anything to please everyone, to avoid disapproval, to avoid making anyone work harder because of us. We also have a difficult time allowing other people to help us because we have a perfectionist attitude. "No one can do my job the way I do it."

It is this group of people, who absorb stress without releasing it, which is most susceptible to developing Fibromyalgia.

Andrew H. Knapp - The Roses and the Oasis

A Scenario

The main cause of Fibromyalgia is stress. Life in modern society is not possible without stress on one or more levels. The schedules of work, of school, of family and of social all add their levels of stress to our individual lives. The clock becomes the enemy, ticking away the minutes as we race to meet schedules, due dates, deadlines and obligations both real and imagined. We wish there were more hours in the day. We stay up later at night to accomplish more of the things that just **have** to get done, cutting into our sleep time which adds to the stress on our body by depriving it of the rest it needs to function properly in our stress filled environment. Lack of sleep becomes chronic as our body struggles to handle its levels of stress. Our body muscles become tense while under stress. The blood shifts from it's normal slightly acid level to a slightly alkaline level causing it to thicken and not function properly. Complete rest is needed to release the tension in our muscles, but deep restful sleep eludes us as we are constantly thinking of our jobs, responsibilities and obligations. Incomplete rest brings on muscle spasms, muscle spasms grow and spread to other muscles, pain becomes manifest in the spreading muscle spasms under the guise of minor aches, fatigue steps in as the body uses large amounts of energy to fight the pain, fatigue becomes heavier and heavier from the combination of fighting pain and

145

not enough complete rest... A scenario of Fibromyalgia has begun. It's never that simple, though.

Some Biology - My Theory

*Author's note: The following is a blending of information from D.C. Jarvis' book, "Folk Medicine", and many other sources and classes which I have studied over the years. It could be called my "theory" of how I believe Fibromyalgia begins.

Fibromyalgia is a slow building, passively developing condition which, little by little, takes hold of one muscle or a set of muscles at a time without the conscious notice of the person being afflicted until it is widespread throughout much of the body and causing a dominating physical pain. Absorbed stress becomes tension in muscles in various places in the body. When a person cannot remove tension in the muscles, this develops into muscle spasms. The muscles become tense like they are ready to fight or run, but since they are not allowed to, they simply hold their readiness. The longer they hold onto this readiness, or emergency readiness mode, without using it or releasing it, the more it becomes a muscle spasm. A muscle spasm can be related to a cramp in that it is involuntary. When the body is in the emergency readiness mode, it is preparing to run or to defend itself. Initially, the blood becomes thinner to be able to get oxygen and nutrients into the muscles making them ready for action. If the body does not take the action it is preparing for, however, the blood will thicken and change from its normal slightly acid level to a slightly alkaline level. When the blood is in an acid level, it flows better, it is more fluid and able to do its work of feeding and cleaning the cells of the body. When the blood is in an alkaline level, it becomes thicker and cannot flow as well as it needs to to get into the finer capillaries of the tissues of the body. The longer the body is in the emergency readiness mode without taking action, the more starved the muscles and tissues will become because of the blood's inability to flow freely. The muscle cells become malnourished which makes them prime for holding onto tension, which I interpret as going into spasm. With each day in which tension is absorbed without being released, the spasm in the muscle grows. As the spasm grows, more of the muscle is involuntarily held tense. As more of the muscle is in spasm, less blood is able to get to the muscle cells. The cells are unable to function properly since they are being deprived of oxygen and nutrients and are unable to remove wastes. This causes a build up of toxins in these cell tissues. This toxin build up irritates the nerves and causes pain in the muscles. As the pain builds up in the muscles, so does the spasm increase. As the spasm increases and fills the muscle, pressure is exerted on the nerve passageways as they pass through that muscle. When a nerve is affected with pressure, it responds by sending a message to the brain. For instance, if there are strong muscle spasms along the splenius capitis, (muscles which follow the length of both sides of the spine) in the middle of the neck, the nerves which leave the spine to go to the hands would be "touched" with pressure from the spasm. This pressure "touch" on the nerve would be sent as a false message to the brain saying that the fingers hurt or are tingling when in reality there is no real or true pain in the fingers at all, only in the place where the muscle spasm "touched" the nerve with pressure. If the body muscles are filled with spasm, then, wherever a nerve passes through, it receives pressure, which gives false information to the brain, which "thinks" there is pain throughout the body, whereas the source of the pain is far from where the brain "thinks" it is. It is at this point where medical science becomes frustrated. X-rays, CT scans, and Magnetic Resonance Imaging (MRI) tests will not show muscle spasm or nerve paths revealing pain sources. Modern medicine has difficulty diagnosing soft-tissue ailments. There is a gauntlet of tests to determine if what is troubling you is something that could be tangible. There are many things which can cause muscle pain and it is important to rule those out before a diagnosis of Fibromyalgia can be certain. There also is a simple test which can be done in the doctor's office to detect the trigger points of Fibromyalgia. Regretfully, though, this test should not be done until after other diseases are ruled out.

Muscle Memory

If there have been traumatic injuries from accidents in a persons past, such as broken bones, sprains and bruises, these places in the body will go into spasm quicker than other parts of the body when under stress because they harbor Trigger Points. At the onset of any accident, muscles try to immobilize the injured part of the body by going into spasm, called splinting, and rushing blood to that area to heal any damaged or broken cells. Long after healing has taken place, these post traumatized muscles will "remember" the former injury reactions when the body is in an emergency readiness mode brought on by a stressful situation. We wonder why certain parts of our bodies, which are unrelated to work activities, act up with pain after a stressful period of time.

Most of us know of people who can tell weather changes are about to occur because a certain ache or pain tells them so. The reason for this is that the blood in the body flows better under a high pressure weather system than it does under a low pressure system. This slightly thicker blood condition is interpreted as a stressful situation by the body. Bad weather always comes under a low pressure system and it is usually cooler temperatures, too. Blood also flows better during warm weather than during cold weather thereby giving the body less stress when the weather is warm. This is why aerobics and heat

151

therapy work against muscle pain by raising body temperature and thinning the blood. Aches and pains will always be more prevalent when the blood does not flow well.

These places of former pain are the first to tell us when our blood is not flowing as it should. They also are a warning for us to take notice when they act up when the weather is good or for no apparent reason. *(Please read D.C. Jarvis' book, "Folk Medicine", to learn how to keep the blood flowing as it should through simple diet adjustments.)

Chronic Fatigue

One scenario which can lead to Fibromyalgia and other physical problems is lack of sleep and rest. Fibromyalgia is said to be caused by a sleeping disorder by some authorities. Indeed, when someone is worried, under stress and/or experiencing hormonal changes, sleep is often hard to come by and then not very deep when it is attained. When someone is under the pressure of work deadlines or coordinating schedules of several family members, sleep is often lost during the process. Sleep which cannot be made up for. When someone is in the emergency readiness mode, sleep is not very complete nor even very possible. When muscles are tense and holding tension, this prevents deep sleep. Someone who is experiencing tension, much of which that person not being conscious of, is spending much energy while struggling to resist it. Without much sleep, this brings on fatigue. The longer in the emergency readiness mode, the longer without good sleep, the deeper the fatigue will be and the more widespread the Fibromyalgia and muscle pain will become due to non-conscious spasms. It is a vicious circle.

If you cannot get good, deep sleep and are not rested upon awakening, look for the sources of stress in your life which are keeping you from the rest you need and try to alleviate them. By the time you notice that you are chronically fatigued, however, your entire body will have been in an emergency readiness mode for a long time before then. Once you are to the noticeable level of chronic fatigue, it will take much more than just sleep to get back to normal. Also, check with your family doctor if you are chronically fatigued to see if there is a tangible cause for it other than stress.

Fear Factor

Once there is muscle pain and fatigue mysteriously evident, another contributing factor steps into the picture. Fear. Fear magnifies the stress levels, the emergency readiness mode, the lack of sleep, and the pain. You are staring into the unknown. After all the tests, there is nothing physically wrong with you. They are probably telling you that "It's all in your head." "You should go back to work." You know how you feel, but they don't believe you. You become desperate. It seems that your whole life is falling apart. In a sense, it is. If something doesn't come along to help you, for you to do, you feel that you may die a slow, agonizing death. Depression is the next step after fear. Depression takes away a person's will.

The fact that you are reading this book shows that you are seeking answers and not falling deeply into depression. Fear may be a motivating factor in your search, but you have not allowed depression to become apathy causing you to lay down and give up. You are out here doing something about your condition. Congratulations. You will not be without reward for your efforts.

Further reading:

I have listed the four books which have helped the most in my journey of overcoming Fibromyalgia. Countless other books, periodicals, doctors, therapists, and educators have helped over the years which are too numerous to hope to remember for this list.

Once you begin your quest for healing, you will find many books which will help along the way. Search not only for answers in dealing with Fibromyalgia, but also for answers for the reasons for what happens. Look for physical, biological, medical, mental, and spiritual answers to help you in understanding your entire person.

Folk Medicine
A Vermont doctor's Guide to Good Health
    by D.C. Jarvis, M.D.
    Holt and Company, 1958
    (many reprints)

Pain Erasure
The Bonnie Prudden Way
    by Bonnie Prudden
    Ballantine Books, 1980

You Gotta Keep Dancin'
        by Tim Hansel
        Lifejourney Books, 1985

Awakening Spirits
a Native American path to inner peace,
healing, and spiritual growth
        by Tom Brown, Jr.
        Berkley Books, 1994

Myotherapists and Massage Therapists:

To find a Myotherapist, Muscle Therapist or Massage Therapist, (be sure they are all certified), first, look in the yellow pages of your local area, then at the library for yellow pages of larger cities nearby, and search the internet. (A web site for Myotherapists is: www.frontiernet.net/~painrel) When you find a therapist, be sure to ask about how they treat Fibromyalgia, Myofascial Pain Syndrome, and if they use Trigger Point Therapy or a form of it when you talk to them. Always remember that **you** are in charge of getting ahead of your condition. Find what works and pursue it. Your freedom is what this is all about.

Andrew H. Knapp - The Roses and the Oasis